Confessions of a Survivor

Confessions
of a
Survivor

Kathleen Barbee

WRITER'S PROOF

ATHENS, GEORGIA

Published by Writer's Proof,
an imprint of Miglior Press

www.migliorpress.com

Cover design by Wendy Garfinkel-Gold
Cover photo by Roger Kirby
Author photo by Marissa Barbee

ISBN 978-0-9822726-5-7

Printed in the United States of America

To Olga Cuyar and Mae Samal Knox

and

in memory of Mark Dragula, my son in law

August 4, 2009

It is the last night of my summer vacation; I had a glorious month off from teaching. Wanting to catch the last few minutes of a decorating show I was enjoying, I pulled the ottoman up to the TV. I began to do a little analysis on myself: "Do I need a mask tonight, or just a good exfoliation?" As I ran my fingers along my jaw bone, I felt a hard lump. "What the heck is this?" I wondered out loud. I ran down my townhouse stairs to my eighteen-year-old daughter's room. "Quick! Feel this for me," I said as I put my face close to her bed.

"That's gross," she said, with typical teenage attitude. It just so happened that I had a doctor's appointment the next day to go over standard blood work. (After three years of procrastination, I had bitten the bullet and had had a physical exam.)

August 5, 2009

Well, I went in for my physical results. No good news. The doctor rattled off the following list: high blood pressure, thyroid off, beginning of osteoporosis, and pointed out I could lose a few pounds. In response to that information, I joked, "Other than that, Mrs. Lincoln, how was the play?" She smiled, and then, oh, one more thing. I asked her, "What is this weird lump?"

All of a sudden the joking was over. As she felt the lump, she seemed very concerned. "You need a C. T. scan ASAP, and I will pray for you."

When does a doctor say "I will pray for you"? It's never good.

She referred me to an ear, nose, and throat (ENT) specialist, Dr. Galin. The results were shocking. "Hard, palpable, discernible mass. Throat area inhomogeneous," whatever that meant. Dr. Galin was beyond somber, navy blue eyes and not a hint of smile.

August 12, 2009

Next step, biopsy. Right before I had to return to work from my summer break, I had to go back to the ENT. This time I had to swallow, through my nostril, a large, black-rubber tube with a "telescope" attached to it.

I began to panic, and Dr. Galin gave me an extra squirt of freeze spray. When he stepped out, waiting for it to take effect, I slid my hand in my purse and took out and then swallowed a five-milligram Valium that I keep for emergencies.

It was not enough! Four suctions, that is four long needles into my neck while I'm in a plastic dental-type chair. My legs stuck to the plastic. (Couldn't they put linen or even paper on this chair?) Shouldn't I have brought someone with me?

As I started to black out, I felt cold liquid rolling down my neck and the front of my dress. "Is that blood?" I asked Dr. Galin.

"It is blood, cells, and gunk," he replied.

Why is there no towel over me and my now-shaking legs? My dress is sliding up as I lay on my side in agony. My eyes fall onto a wall of brochures that read, in bold black and red letters "You Have Head and Neck Cancer, Now What?" I am reciting my act of contrition in my head over and over when the perky young nurse says to me, "I love your shoes!"

Four vials of "gunk" are sent to the lab. Now I just wait.

August 26, 2009

I started my new class. Everyone wanted to know why my neck was in bandages. I told a white lie: "I had something removed."

This seems like a great group of students.

August 27, 2009
2:00 a.m.

Today I found out I have cancer. I must be in shock because I am wide awake, no naps, no coffee, just pure adrenaline. I have a malignant lump on my neck that has metastasized. The good news is my kids are rallying around me. [See "About My Kids," p. 106.]

I have been lonely and no one knew. Today was like a dream come true. Gina, my oldest, (often critical) daughter drove over with the [her] kids to see Grandmom. I baked cookies; Marissa, the eighteen-year old, actually had dinner cooking on the stove for us! We all hugged, cried, and my son Ryan called me twice in one day! (He can go months without a word.) Ever since I have been awaiting my results, Ryan calls faithfully. Rachel, one of my grown adopted kids, called from Georgia and sent her love. My oldest son, George, has been in constant touch from the hospital where he is a department head. He wants me to fax all my records up to him tomorrow. I feel so loved.

My faith is so strong, and I am okay. Hopefully, when I am poked and prodded in the hospital this weekend, I can take it. They need to find where my cancer is coming from.

I'm going to call everyone I love. Why should I hold back anymore? I want to see people! I want to experience as much life as I possibly can, God willing!

August 29, 2009
Saturday, 6:00 a.m.

I am showered, eye make-up on, and hair blown out. I am getting ready to go get my P. E. T. scan. This will pinpoint the primary cancer location. I had to fast except for protein and black coffee. I am starting this thing at five feet five inches and a size twelve. I admit I am a little too curvy.

Yesterday, after being asked all day by co-workers about my neck bandages, I told a couple of people in the next building to mine, while I was making some copies, the truth about the biopsy. They were so kind.

Unfortunately, by the end of the day, word had spread and everyone on campus, it seemed, "just happened" to be in my office area. One co-worker, Juana, who never gives me the time of day, gave me a beautiful chocolate-covered strawberry. On this special diet, of course, I could not enjoy it, but I know people mean well. They just freak out and act like "too close for comfort."

The pathology report was faxed to George, and he emailed me: "Mom, you are the strongest woman I have ever met, you have never given up on anything, and why should this cancer fight be any different?" What a compliment from my oldest son!

Later

I went to dinner with a nice guy named Jim recently, and we keep in touch by email. I was lying on my sofa trying to recuperate from the quadruple biopsy. On my laptop came the funniest video—from Jim. It was an episode of *Who Wants to Be a Millionaire*. The question was "what is larger? The moon, a peanut, or an elephant?" After ten excruciating minutes, during which the contestant used her fifty-fifty poll of the audience and her "phone a friend" and with no other options left, she says "elephant." I laughed so hard, I was crying. When I messaged back, I told Jim his timing was perfect and let him know what was going on with me. He was so sweet and supportive. Now we are chatting again, and it's a good thing.

Still Later

Marissa has a date, and I do not want to be home alone. So, Jim is stopping by. As it turns out, my friend Jill and her boyfriend, Dennis, are also stopping by.

Midnight

Well, it turned into an impromptu dinner party. Me, the ultimate planner, had to wing it! My friend Patricia came by bearing gifts. With everyone sharing food and laughter, it was a wonderful night. I had given Marissa my last twenty dollars before she went out, and by the grace of God my dear friends gave me gas and grocery gift cards. My car was on empty. Looks like we will be okay.

PET-Scan Day

I am secretly taking a five milligram Valium right before my scan, due to my claustrophobia. My girls, Marissa and Gina, hopefully, will support each other and me. It hasn't always been a picnic with all the different personalities.

Now I am curious! Where the hell is the cancer coming from? Just for today, I feel blessed by so many people. Made only one call, to my friend Nicki. She lost her twenty-four-year-old daughter to colon cancer. This beautiful girl was a third-year medical student, who was repeatedly misdiagnosed until it was way too late. I didn't want to add to Nicki's burden.

However, after losing a child, nothing compares. So, I gave her the task of calling two mutual girlfriends. I neglected all my friends all summer. If this doesn't get me off the hook, nothing will! Now I wonder, all that reflective time by myself in the ocean, was it my spiritual preparation?

August 30, 2009
Saturday, 11:00 p.m.

The PET scan felt like I was stuck on Disney's "It's a Small World After All." It was a ride that moves slowly through a dark tunnel, then it jerks back in the opposite direction. Thirty-five minutes of this. I squeezed my eyes shut and envisioned all the little dolls lined up singing "It's a small world after all." Then my head was put into a vice. (A "mammogram" of the skull, it lasted another fifteen minutes.)

For the treatment, after they insert the IV, you are placed in a room with other sick people. Everyone is lying in semi-darkness on recliners. It is about forty degrees in there. The walls are puke green, and there is no art work or music. You are told that you are not allowed to move or talk. It hit me like a ton of bricks. It has only been a couple of days since my diagnosis. This is real. Too real. I am one of these sick people.

Earlier our plans fell through. Gina wanted to bring all three grandkids. Can you imagine three unruly kids sitting still for almost three hours? Marissa was gracious enough to stay with the kids at their home. They told Gina to just drop me off as it was a minimum of two and a half hours. My technician was so gentle and kind. Karen chattered away and helped distract me. God bless her.

After everything was over, Marissa and I hightailed it out of Gina's. We went to lunch at Panera Bread. Rissy began to cry a little bit. We just held each others hands over the soup and sandwiches. I guess she realizes Mom's not so bad to have around.

When I got home, I went online. The first thing I Googled was lung cancer, even though I never smoked. I just don't know where it is coming from. The information was very sobering, to say the least.

Marissa had a date. I called both ex-husbands, and one returned my call. Richard, Marissa's dad. When I got done with my spiel about my tumor and my testing, including all the trauma, Richard says, "Kath, so sorry about Ted Kennedy's passing."

"Hello! What about my diagnosis? Just because I'm from Boston— we aren't related to the Kennedys!" We both started laughing, and it was wonderful. Richard was very sweet to me. My one request was that he call Marissa more often and get more involved in her life. I will be very busy fighting this demon, I told him, and she will need her dad. He agreed.

August 30, 2009
Sunday, 9:30 p.m.

Just ate an entire container of Chunky Monkey. I don't want to look back in a few months and say, "Why didn't I indulge when I could." Today I was in Target, and I had a mini anxiety attack.

Looking into the mirror in the cosmetic department, I caught a glimpse of my bandaged neck. It hit me. Cancer. I looked at all the happy people, families, grandparents, and then the teenaged girls trying on eyeshadow. I felt sick. My heart started racing. I still had a Valium in my purse from the first biopsy. In the perfume aisle, I popped one in my mouth. Then I spent $240.00 on crazy things, like new eye liner and gold eye shadow.

Later, Rachel called. She is my middle daughter I handpicked from Catholic Social Services, when she was ten years old. She had been in the foster system most of her life. She has had her problems but has a big heart. She had an abnormal Pap test and needed a follow-up biopsy. We wished each other well, and both of us broke down and cried a bit.

When I got off the phone, I cleaned the whole garage, did the litter box, and caught up with the laundry. Next a made a pot of homemade soup. Then I crashed; my body said "enough!"

September 1, 2009

Been up since 4:30 a.m. Folded three loads of laundry, washed all the tile floors, brushed the cat, showered and shampooed, and packed for the hospital. Marissa did not come home last night.

She called and said she needed her boyfriend Nick's support. I guess it's me and the cat for my support. Oh, well, I can move about the house and make as much noise as I want.

Yesterday was a whirlwind of meetings, lectures, and organizing my lesson plans for my substitute teacher. The doctor called me at work to remind me to pick up my film on DVD for the hospital. My pre-op blood work was scheduled for 4:00 p.m. It took two more hours and several more tests.

I dragged myself home, and there was no dinner. I know Marissa is just eighteen, but I had a week's worth of groceries in the fridge, and we had planned our menus in advance, over the weekend. Day one [score], zero.

I just needed her to step up. We had words. Then I cooked for us. Then we cleaned up together and went to buy magazines for the hospital.

Thank God my sister Donna is coming on Friday from Boston. I feel so alone.

Later, Same Day

Being wheeled into OR now. All I can say is "in Jesus' name."

September 1, 2009
Night time

Fact findings of the exploratory were that the cancer is confined to my neck and throat area. The primary site is way in back of my tongue. It is so far back it cannot be removed. It is the size of a grape. They can try to shrink it with simultaneous radiation and chemotherapy. The hard mass on the side of my throat is from the first site.

The good news was no vital organs are involved. There is a good chance I could kill this thing, but it will be grueling. I need to be seen by the oncologist ASAP.

Everyone was wonderful! How great are these OR nurses and surgical techs. They cocooned me in heated blankets and love. This morning I got on my knees and asked God "to guide the surgeon's hands," and he did. My pain is minimal with the meds, and I only needed one dose of pain mediation.

Marissa stepped up to the plate. She made stuffed ravioli with wild mushrooms and Alfredo sauce. She tossed a fresh salad, and after twenty-four hours of fasting, I ate every bite!

The anti-nausea drugs worked, and I held the dinner down. Then a glorious nap. So I enjoyed two of the gifts God gave us: the ability to rest our weary bones and enjoy good food.

Maybe I am in denial. After all, it is still a cancer diagnosis, but *not* a life sentence.

Feeling loved is new for me. Not since I was married have I felt nurtured. My girls Gina and Rissy called twenty loving close friends for me. My son-in-law came with my grandson Mac, and they made me laugh. Another gift from God: laughter.

September 2, 2009

Last night I was in my own bed, savoring every bit of life I have been granted. A comfortable mattress, my hand-stitched quilt from my sister Donna, and on the wall my wooden crucifix from my grandmother's casket. All my favorite books and Bible are within easy reach.

Then when I got to Dr. Feinstein's office, the reality set in. He phoned me and simply said, "the sooner, the better." His urgency was beyond scary, but at 10:00 a.m. there I was, sitting on his examining table. Now that I know how these things roll, I asked

DeeAnn, my friend and former business partner, to drive me. She was busy in the morning, so Rissy stepped in. I hope she can handle it. DeeAnn will come by later, when I see the radiologist at 3:00 p.m. Okay, we have a plan.

On the way to Dr. Feinstein's, Marissa snapped at me and was complaining that her boyfriend was an "ass" for not comforting her enough with "her mother dying."

"Gee, thanks," I snapped back. "Can I at least *try* to kick this thing?"

* * * * *

Dr. Feinstein pulled no punches. "You have two things going for you: you have ten or fifteen extra pounds and clear lungs from never smoking. It looks like fifty-fifty."

My co-worker Larry came by the house for tea. He gave me a fifty-dollar Publix gift card for groceries. That's about as sentimental and close to Hallmark as it gets for him; I sure appreciated his thoughtfulness.

As we had tea and pastries, he caught me up on work gossip. Just a couple of days out of work, and I feel so out of the loop. It was a wonderful two hours of catching up on the latest.

My dear sister Donna is flying in on Friday. I can't wait! The boys—my sons George and Ryan and my grandson Evan—are planning a trip down from Gainesville.. Gina has been calling; everyone is so loving to me. Who knew?

On exploratory day at the hospital, my son-in-law Mark came right out and asked Dr. Galin, "how long does she have?" (You have to love him; he's clueless.) Poor Dr. Galin just froze. Nothing subtle about Mark. Subtle as a train wreck!

Tonight my throat hurts. I made homemade chili—okay, not the best choice. I already lost three pounds. Dr. Feinstein said ten more lost and I'll have to get a feeding tube, ugh. Tomorrow starts chemotherapy and radiation. Both! This is surreal.

September 3, 2009
3:00 a.m.

Okay. Now I am a bit shaky. Marissa slept at Nick's. ("Because she is eighteen and an adult now," according to her.)

It isn't in me to argue with her at this stage of the game. So as I wander the house, it hits me: cancer cells are multiplying while I sleep, also while I walk about and twenty-four hours a day.

I scrambled an egg, put on TV. Ironically, it was an old Cosby show, rerun, about Theo, the oldest son, trying to come to terms with his buddy's cancer! His closest pal was in the hospital, and it was so well done, I laughed out loud and also cried my eyes out.

I do feel God "allowed me" to get this cancer as a punishment for every lousy, unkind thing I ever said to anyone. For any hurtful words, I probably deserved it. Even though I have worked on being kinder for the last twenty years, I admit the first twenty I was self-centered. I am still working on myself and my spirituality daily. Never would I say "why me?" Why not me? I am so flawed, and I don't get a free pass in this life.

Okay. Now my neck looks like I swallowed two gerbils. Finding turtlenecks in South Florida is like finding a lemonade stand in

New England in winter. I'm looking for the sleeveless kind in a hurry and shortly my neck will look like a bag of kittens.

Must ask my dear sister Donna to tell my other siblings—Walter, sister Pat, and Tom—that it breaks my heart to make anyone worry. It isn't that we are exceptionally close, this motley-crew family of mine; however, it isn't fun news to have to share.

Can I overcome this? I don't know. I am so tired; I feel beaten up by life already. Where is David, my husband of seventeen years? Even Marissa's dad, Richard, came through for me. Even with his alcoholism, he has such an open heart. Dave has always been so stingy with his heart; why should he be different now? It still hurts me, and I still miss married life with him.

My mom awaits me, my loving grandparents. Two dear girlfriends, Barbara W. and Barbara H., both breast cancer. My seventeen-year-old baby sitter, Kim (car wreck), my student Chelsea, eighteen (motorcycle). My twenty-one-year-old nephew (gun), and my wonderful dad. My favorite cousin, Bobby, dropped dead at forty, and on and on. But how I love the living! My precious babies. Okay. Here come the tears.

September 4, 2009

Yesterday was by far one of the worst, most-sobering days of my life. I asked DeeAnn to drive me to the oncologist. Thank God I was not alone.

Here is Dr. Feinstein's plan: radiation five times a week, chemotherapy one six-hour day per week. So one day a week is a double whammy. If I lose ten more pounds, I get the feeding tube, no questions asked, no option. If I lose my ability to breathe on my own, I will get a tracheotomy. Even if I survive, I may lose my ability to speak or swallow. With the most aggressive treatment, my odds are fifty-fifty.

Second choice, we could go in the hospital tomorrow, and he could amputate my tongue and eliminate all tumors completely. He says most people elect the chemo-radiation route. Gee, wonder why? So let's go with plan one. Ah. . .okay.

The visit went on and on. Several vials of blood later, DeeAnn looked like she was going to pass out. We walked out of there like two zombies, holding hands. The silence was deafening on the walk to the car.

Later On. Same Day.

Donna arrives from Boston tomorrow. Hopefully, so will George, Evan, and Ryan from Gainesville. Help is on the way! I am on a wing and a prayer, and I still have to see the radiologist tomorrow. Alone!

September 4, 2009
Midnight

Just climbed into my clean bed in my new PJs from my sister. Love is the greatest healer. Donna almost did not make it; she got bumped in New York on her connecting flight. She left me a message saying she *would not* be arriving at 3:00 p.m. I was just devastated.

After a long morning at the radiologist, I came crawling in the door at lunch time. I forced myself to try to eat something, as Dr. Bushbaum was even more adamant about getting a feeding tube into me. He explained the radiation would make it very difficult, if not impossible, to swallow. How frightening is that? For two and a half hours, we went over every step of treatment. He gave me the same odds as Dr. Feinstein had, fifty-fifty chance of being able to eradicate the cancer. I feel like I am in a dream. Who can hear these horrible realities and continue to function? I guess I can. And I will.

Donna finally made it. What a breath of fresh air! To have her step off the plane: Somebody loves me. She was rerouted to Fort Lauderdale and during rush hour no less! (Marissa opted not to go with me. I was ready to snap when she said, "I just want to chill." I know she is cranky and selfish, but also hurting.) I hope Donna can help heal Marissa while she is here. She has her work cut out for her. Thanks be to God, I have a family.

September 5, 2009
Saturday 10:30 a.m.

It was wonderful to have Donna and George here this morning. We got so much accomplished. We organized a list of family and friends to help out. Once treatment begins, I will need someone to drive me. Donna bought a large white board for the kitchen, and we had George hang it up for scheduling. I told her the oncologist said there has to be one general for the family. She appointed herself. When George (six feet, two inches) arrived, he teased Donna, all of five feet, of having a Napoleon complex. George did all the heavy work for us. I felt so loved by my oldest son and Sisterbelle. When Marissa came home, we all sat in the living room and had a heart-to-heart talk with her about the next few weeks and what each of us could do to endure. She cried and let it all out. We had a beautiful group hug, and then Marissa broke the mood by saying, "Is this an intervention?" We all laughed through our tears.

Later on I was able to make a pot of homemade soup and pick up some fresh French bread for Gina and Mark's house. Gina was so excited to see her brother as she had only expected Aunt Donna to be with us. We ate in the dining room with all the children. What a glorious family time it was!

As we all laughed, I felt so blessed to have their love and support. The kids ran around while the adults lingered at the table. There was something so old fashioned, sitting around that large, round table. It was like stepping back in time. Laughter was my medicine tonight.

* * * * *

Now it is midnight, and I am back home in bed. I have an unbearable earache on the left tumor side of my head. I noticed they are growing very fast. The one in my throat is less visible from the outside, but it makes me choke. Eating is getting more difficult. I am praying for the strength to get though this. Tomorrow my family leaves, and I know I will feel lonely again. Hopefully they return soon.

Marissa acts angry at me for getting sick. I guess it isn't what you expect at eighteen, the possibility of losing a parent. So very sorry.

September 6, 2009
Sunday
5:00 p.m.

Alone for the first time in days. Not a good thing.

September 10, 2009
Thursday
5:30 a.m.

Very busy couple of days, trying to cover all my bases, barely keeping my head above water. Yesterday I stopped by the college to see about my medical leave. First of all, they moved HR across campus. (Why would I expect a sign up? Why would they have adequate parking spaces available?) I felt so weak, zig-zagging through the quads. Meanwhile, rowdy students were having some type of music festival. How surreal was this, sweating, losing my breath, and trying to dodge the crowd in my high heels.

After fifteen minutes of hiking across campus, I found it. Dr. Ellen is our top HR person and just a lovely person, inside and out. The first thing she did was hug me tightly. Then she said all the right things. She introduced me to her assistant. She led me to a small, windowless, dingy room, and I began to feel panic. The room had 1970's paneling and a flickering fluorescent light. An old round kitchen set sat in the center of the room. She was a very overweight woman with a beet-red face and no smile. She looked old, yet she was probably only thirty-five or forty. I have never given a thought to my benefits, except when half of Marissa's braces were covered. Now I was about to find out, it is like trying to cash out your own CD's early. They aren't going to let you have what's yours.

We went round and round. The bottom line was that when my vacation time runs out, I will have a two-month gap with no pay. That's four paychecks! I would be about four grand in the hole. I explained that I was a one-income household. Her eyes stayed ice cold. "So am I," she stated.

"I have an eighteen year old who could never run the household on her part-time job," I said. Poker faced, she would not budge. She slid the medical-leave forms across the table to me; I slid them back. "No way can I survive without eight weeks of salary," I told her.

It was like being in an interrogation room with someone trying to get me to sign a confession. My voice cracked, and my eyes welled up. Now I feel sick, hot and frightened and claustrophobic, all at once. "Do you know what type of cancer I have?" I asked her, my voice rising.

"Yes," she said, "that is how my father died." She showed no emotion.

Oh, my God. I got it. Good cop, bad cop. The college would lose money if more professors took their leave. How I got up and walked out, I don't know. I stuffed the unsigned forms in my purse and just bolted.

Driving across campus to my building, I tried to get my composure. I had some thank-you notes to distribute. Looks like my substitute was doing okay. My office was not disturbed. My desk still had its mementos and photos. It meant so very much to me to see my things left in place. My white smock was still across my office chair, my favorite artwork still up, and even my plant looked happy.

I sat and had coffee with my co-workers. How wonderful is this. To feel normal, even for an hour. All the faces of students and friends offering me emotional support meant so much. A few people tried to pool their own leave time for me, but they were refused. Looks like there isn't much help provided. Just then a "higher up" popped in to say, "Work from home on your computer. Whatever you do, do not sign the papers for leave." If you pop in when you can, your hours will be good. I'm sure you have lots of prep work and research for future classes." God blessed me once more, and I dodged a bullet.

10:00 p.m.

My eyes are burning; I am so weak. Today I ran a fever, my white count was way off, and I found out I've lost three more pounds. I had to promise Dr. Feinstein if the weight went down any more, I would get the tube. No more excuses.

For now, I am okay. My chemo was ordered; there was a problem with my Blue Cross paying for it. They have their own distributor where it is a few dollars cheaper than where Dr. Feinstein orders his. Mine has to be specially mailed by itself. I walked out of the oncologist's office depressed.

Before I left I said to the doctor, "Would you please show me where the chemo room is?" He did not look too happy. As we walked by the comfy waiting room chairs and the fish tanks, I could see, way in the back, a room like a scene in a Civil War movie, *The Living Dead*. That's all I could think. A big, square box of a room with IV drips hanging near each soulless face. Under thin, white blankets in semi-reclining chairs, all ages and all types of people lay down together. A few sad-looking relatives sat on straight-back chairs beside some of them.

"This is so depressing," I could not help but say.

Dr. Feinstein looked surprised. "Look, we have a TV, over there in the corner," he proudly announced.

"I have one of those at home," I glumly replied. How strange was that? My family got their first TV in the 1940's, a TV with a remote control in 1956, and a color TV in 1965. It was hardly a new invention.

Walking out, I was hit by rain from a torrential downpour. No warning, no umbrella, all my medical papers in an open tote bag. I slumped down and tried not to cry. I looked at my phone. Missed calls. One was Jim. "Call me anytime for anything," was his message. I called him back. Chit chat. Then I braved the rain, got to my car, and then made it to a nearby bagel shop.

The air conditioning was freezing cold, and I was soaking wet. I was sipping hot coffee when my phone rang. Jim. "Do you want to see a movie with me?" he asked.

"Yes!" It was a life line, and I was grabbing it. Rushing home to change, I dropped some bagels off to Marissa and her girlfriend who stayed over. Within twenty minutes I pulled up to the theatre. Here was Jim under an umbrella with two tickets to see *Inglourious Basterds* with Brad Pitt.

Just what the doctor ordered. Brad Pitt showed me how much people endured in the Holocaust. More than any human should ever have to. I was ashamed of myself for being such a wimp about enduring two months of chemo. Big deal. Suck it up and just do it.

* * * * *

That evening, Marissa and I had a social-worker meeting with "Palmaire"; her name sounded like an airline. She was a nice-enough girl, but totally overwhelmed by our flood of tears. Surely we can't be the only family going through this that breaks down. Two boxes of tissues later, we stumbled out of there.

Bottom line, we process differently. I jump in and plan and organize, then delegate. Rissy processes much more slowly as she adjusts to each new bit of information, slowly.

* * * * *

We must respect that we are both hurting. Oh, my God, I really do have cancer. I'm drained. Several loving messages awaited me, but I just went to bed and Marissa went to Nick's house.

My last thought of the day—remember all those Jewish families in the movie losing all their loved ones, the suffering and starvation. It went on daily, sometimes for years. What a drop in the bucket two months of treatment is. "Buck up and be strong," I tell myself. Imagine if I had said "no" to Jim? His movie invitation gave me the courage I surely needed.

September 11, 2009

No word from David. How can you be married to someone for almost eighteen years and then nothing? It still hurts.

Nine-eleven. How many hearts are still broken from that date? Everyone else's courage dealing with their pain gives me strength to keep going.

The intense pain woke me up. The earache on the left side is horrendous. My head is on fire.

Stupid worries go through my head. Who will dust my living room when I'm out of it? Who will clean my bathroom when the smell of cleaning products makes me sick?

Should I spend $100.00 to have Marissa's carpet cleaned? Does it even matter? Should I ask my sons to do it, when they visit?

Randomly I say to myself during the day, "I have cancer." I'm still making a recovery plan, but I have lots of paperwork to get straightened out.

I was modifying my mortgage payment; there is so much to do and get faxed off.

What if I cause us to lose our home? I need some help. I am afraid to bother anyone.

9:00 p.m.

Today has been very emotional for me. I haven't been able to even read any material or view any documentaries about 9/11. With that said, I got through the day and night. I organized all my banking paperwork. Then I went in person. My banker, Angela, is also a friend. When she saw me, looking thin and pale, she was devastated. She gave me some numbers of people who could possibly help me moderate my mortgage.

Then I swung by work. I did a bit of paperwork and felt normal. It was great. I could tell that my substitute, Christina, was doing a good job. My students came by for hugs, and it fed my soul.

Unfortunately, I overdid it. I phoned Marissa to make dinner plans. I told her to defrost some steak, and her friend Alex joined us. Every one of my doctors is stressing protein at every meal. The girls went out after dinner; ten minutes later they called, dead battery. I had no energy left to help them. I had Chardonnay with dinner, and it did me in. My cancer cells are saying "what the?" I am not who I was, and I have new limitations.

A niece I haven't seen or spoken to in years called. Her name is Angela. At first, I thought it was my banker. She heard I was sick and wanted to tell me she modeled herself after me as a wife and mother. She said she would have never made it through child-hood without me. (Her mom, my older sister, Pat, had some prob-lems.) Angela said she learned how to cook and be a good mom from me. What an honor to receive that message. I never knew I was her mentor.

September 12, 2009
Saturday
3:30 p.m.

My head hurts. I took a Valium for stress. Marissa has been spend-ing more nights at Nick's. She has called me repeatedly to say she will meet up with me, to help with groceries, errands, etc. Then she will move the meeting time ahead. Now she phoned me to say she will be later getting home as they are helping Nick's mom do "stuff" around the house and move things for her.

Okay. I unload a case of water, all the groceries, and heavy cat litter by myself. No problem. Then I made some lunch, a Boost shake, trying to add some calories. It is becoming difficult to keep my weight up. Finally, I passed out on the sofa for a much-need-ed nap. My phone kept waking me: Ananda, my ex-daughter-in-law whom I love like a daughter called, and then Gina checks in. Finally DeeAnn calls to insist on accompanying me to my first chemo and to give Marissa moral support. All supportive, loving calls.

I was still trying to rest when Marissa and Nick came in. Big bear hug from Nick (okay, let go, still alive, getting awkward). Then

Nick charges Marissa's dead battery again and proceeds to fix them a late lunch.

"Mom, can we talk?" Marissa asks me.

"Okay," I say, trying to lighten the mood, "just don't tell me you're pregnant."

"No, but I need a passport. Nick's mom and her boyfriend invited me to Mexico over the weekend of October 31st. I will also need a little spending money. What do you think?"

I stared at her as if I had never seen her in my life. "Until I have my first chemo, I have no idea how I will feel. What if I can't even walk to the bathroom without help? That would be a problem."

"Okay, then," she replied. "I'll ask George and Kendra (my son and oldest granddaughter) to come stay with you."

I was incredulous. "Whatever you want to do, Marissa, but before I even endure one chemo or radiation treatment, I will not give you my blessing on this trip, *out of the country*!"

She glared at me. "Why do you have to be such a bitch about it?"

"Well, let's see," I said. "If Nick's mom got diagnosed with MS, I might not pick up the phone and invite Nick to Disney World!"

Just then my phone rang. It was Donna. I didn't hold back *at all*. I relayed the whole conversation. Marissa raised her voice and said I was trying to make her look bad, and it was all my fault! I replied that in the last few days I have paid your cell-phone bill, your prescription, and bought a tire for your car. I have given you gas money and *now you need a passport and spending money?*" I really lost it then. "I can't even afford to pick up my anti-nausea pre-scription for chemo until my paycheck goes in on Monday, and you need play money?"

She went storming downstairs and then phoned me to continue the argument.

My blood pressure sky rocketed; I feel sick to my stomach. All I can think is my cancer cells love this turmoil, so they can multiply faster and faster.

I may have to ask her to leave. She has not been able to give me much support. If it is too much to expect from an eighteen-year-old, then just go! I want to live! I need people in my life to help me, not add more stress to me.

9:00 p.m.

Knock-down, drag-out, emotional fight with Rissy. Lots of tears (both of us), screaming (her), and just a rotten, bottom-of-the-barrel night. Now the special dinner I made, from the dietician's "cancer-menu" list is stuck in my chest. The radiologist set up an appointment for me with the dietician/nutritionist. It is sup-posed to teach me how "not feed the cancer cells," but keep the weight up. My eyes are puffy from crying. It is too much for both of us. I'm sad, lonely, and afraid. I'm also angry Marissa can't em-pathize with what I'm dealing with. Now she is getting ready to go to Nick's again. I asked her not to and let him come by here after he gets out of work. No, she can't relax here, she told me. She is angry that I need her.

I had four missed calls while I was downstairs going through Fam-ily Drama 101. Ryan, Donna, Patty, and Gayle all called to check in on me. I might ask Patty to sleep over tomorrow night, if I feel this lonely. Gayle is coming by for tea at two tomorrow also.

We need help!

September 13, 2009
Sunday
6:00 a.m.

Swollen eyes, earaches, and a trip to hell and back. There was too much release of emotion yesterday, and I feel ill. It is healthy for us to get it out but not all at once.

When I went down to the garage to get the cat, I was surprised to see Nick sprawled across Marissa's floor, sound asleep. Now they will "chill," as they say, until noon.

Cancer threw our lives into a frenzy. I was very content and happy to have a good work week, a nice dinner, and a new book. Bobbing in the waves all summer, saying my prayers of gratitude, I knew the other shoe would drop. I was so "high" on life. All by myself with a little cooler and some reading material, I would grab my towel and rush to the beach like a little kid. If I am strong enough, I will try to drive out to the beach later.

What a thrill I would get in South Florida when the sun goes down in summer. The water turns silver. The waves reflect the sunset. I would feel I was swimming in God's jewelry box.

This morning I had a brainstorm: to get extra calories, I put the "adult formula" (that is disgusting) in my coffee. Not too bad!

If I make it to the other side of this, to health again, I will help other cancer patients. Nobody addresses the sorrow and shock. I imagine that no matter what part of the body it strikes, you say "why there?"

Here I am, four natural childbirths (well, one C-section) and pushing sixty. Do I need my uterus? No. Do I need my ovaries? No. Clean and cancer free. Do I need these double-D breasts? No, I live like a nun. It has been fifteen years since I have had a husband, and I have chosen not to have a boyfriend while Marissa is still home. My mammograms are perfect. Now do I need my neck? Yes, to hold my head up. My tongue? Yes, to eat and speak. Maybe even to kiss someone again someday.

I'm afraid if I got to church, I will begin to cry and make a fool of myself. I put Pastor Joel Osteen on TV and get a fix of positivity and my spiritual food each Sunday.

Lessons of the Week

1. Don't take on too much at one time

2. Plan rest time ahead

3. When people say "what can I do for you," get my courage up to say what I need, whether it's "could you pick up some paper towels?" or "I need cat food for Simbah. (Otherwise, I end up with stuffed animals and funereal flower arrangements all over the house!)

When Patricia showed up, she had twenty rolls of toilet paper, a gas card, and a Publix grocery card for us! She threw in some scandal magazines. Common sense is a wonderful thing.

8:30 p.m.

Roller-coaster day. Rough start. First, Marissa and I had words over something insane. She was having her morning coffee, watching a show on China. I plopped down on the sofa next to her. "Isn't China so beautiful," she said. "I want to go there some day."

Without thinking, I said, "It's one of the dirtiest places in the world, overcrowded and the water is filthy!" I don't know why I was so negative, but I hit a nerve, we were off!

"Why can't you be supportive?" she wailed. "I want to travel and see the world some day," and on and on.

"I just want to live through Christmas," I said.

Later, I took a ride to Barnes and Noble and just slowed down. I called Marissa and apologized, and we made dinner plans together.

Then my well-meaning, overbearing friend Gayle came by. We had tea and cookies. (I sent a package of cookies to her kids.) She has opinions on absolutely everything: my doctors, my medicine, my diet, and on and on. Now I do appreciate the care; however, after four cups of tea and a pounding headache, I had to almost push her out the door.

Glorious fifteen-minute nap before Marissa was back. I made us a nice dinner. I was actually hungry. What a blessing! Marissa offered to give me a back massage, and I took her up on it. It was lovely!

Now I'm in my PJs, and Dr. Craig just called to check on me. I'm feeling a little more grounded tonight.

Earlier today, a stranger gave me the finger in traffic. I wanted to roll down the window and yell "I have cancer; give me a break!"

My regular deli lady at the market actually stepped away from me when I told her I have cancer. It's not contagious!

September 16, 2009
Tuesday

Life is better! Sunday, Gayle called and asked what shoe size I wear. I said eight, and she actually said "Oh, too bad. I'm a ten. I would love your shoe collection!" Joke or not, I am fighting for my life. Just not funny. (I'm glad she has big feet!) I am going to have a code on my call list, who *not* to let visit when I'm down and out.

So why is life better? Monday night Patricia came over and made bruschetta, Marissa had her girlfriend Alex over and they made a fresh salad. I made eggplant parmesan, and we just had a good time. Marissa broke up with Nick *again*, and today they made up. I need to remove myself from their drama to focus on my health.

Jim called me. It is as though I asked the Make a Wish Foundation for a comforting man next to me. Last night, we had snacks and wine on my sofa. We laughed and talked until one a.m.!

I love life! What have I been afraid of? My sister Donna checks on me daily by phone. George, too, checks in often. He called last night while Jim was here, and I said, "I have company."

"Why," he joked, "do you mean a 'gentleman caller'?"

So funny and sweet. Ryan also checks in daily. My sister Pat, from

Boston, sent me a chocolate-covered fruit bouquet. I feel cared for, and it's been a long time.

I stopped by my campus; I was just in the way. The transition from career professional to vulnerable patient is a shock!

Yesterday morning I had to go to the dentist to have a mouth guard made. They felt so bad they only charged me the lab fee. I saved $150.00. Small blessings I am grateful for.

A stranger named Jim (not my Jim) called to say he was an eight-year survivor from neck and tongue cancer. He gave me some hope; he was a neighbor of my dear friend Heidi, who gave him my number.

So I am seeing the best of mankind and the worst. Simultaneously! God's plan for me is perfect, and even with this cancer growing, I have faith life will get better. My spirits are back up. I have now faced death and choose life.

September 17, 2009
Wednesday
11:00 p.m.

I went from the most beautiful lunch on the ocean with Marissa today to the depths of despair. I made a mistake by calling that cancer-survivor, Jim, back. I cannot even write the horrid things he said to me as I am still in shock. I may not be able to get this out of my head. Serious prayers are needed. Soon, he said, I will not be able to eat one bite or even use the bathroom! He spent 118 days in the hospital (he counted), and now eight years later he is alive. It was just too graphic for me, and I am now paralyzed with fear.

Just in case I don't make it, I'm going to write my loved ones a letter each.

September 18, 2009
Thursday

Had my meltdown today. I cried and yelled at a little old Spanish lady at the grocery store.

First, I had a crappy evening. Jim sent me a Carol King song, "You've Got a Friend," on the computer. That is the bittersweet kind of thing to push someone over the edge. And my friend Margaret cancelled my healing session that I surely needed.

My sister Donna called to check on me, and I missed it. I was down in the garage doing laundry. My only contact with the world today was this cancer survivor telling me I would be "swallowing razor blades every day."

Today I pushed myself to get out early to mail those papers to the cancer center for any kind of help. After copying twenty different forms at Office Depot, they said I could not mail them to a post-office box; I needed a physical address. When I finally got hold of the lady on the phone, she said, "We don't give out our address."

It isn't an abortion clinic; it's supposed to be a resource center for cancer patients! The clerk at Office Depot felt sorry for me and did not charge me for the oversized envelope. Next I went to the neighborhood mail center. Why do I feel a need to tell everyone I am sick? It is not comfortable for people to be put on the spot, but I can't shut up.

I got the package off, and my dentist called my cell phone. More good news. He had a phone conference with my radiologist and told me my salivary glands will all be destroyed, and I need another prescription, basically for synthetic spit. Sounds disgusting, but I agreed to go in tomorrow for my seminar—"Living with Dry Mouth"—and to have a special mouth tray made (in the event I live, I will need it).

In the grocery store I filled my cart like a condemned woman. I can still eat! I may as well appreciate the ability to make my own saliva. Every possible food I thought the kids would enjoy this weekend, I threw in, plus beer and wine. Even Simbah got three kinds of gourmet food.

Now it hit me: I'm overtired, sweaty, and feeling sad. I met a nice lady by the blood-pressure machine. She wore a crucifix, so I took that as a sign to tell yet another stranger my diagnosis. Donna called my cell, and I asked her this question: "how many packages of cookies make it an obsession?"

After a pause, she said, "three," and I responded, "I'm in trouble."

By the time I dragged myself to the register, I was shaky. Two hundred dollars later, I turned to leave with my overstuffed cart. Every time I'm in a supermarket, it seems to me, I am asked "do you need some help with that?" One onion and a newspaper, and, still, they ask. Now I am ready to hit the floor, with a container of kitty litter about to fall out, eggs precariously balanced on the case of beer: nothing! Not even a thank you.

"I need help," I said.

The store employee looked at me blankly and said, "You do?"

"Yes. Please."

Now she took the cart from me and walked out of the store. She went in the opposite direction of where my car was parked. "I'm looking for a gray Celica on the other side," I told her. No response. Up one row and down another, with me trying to keep up with her. Finally, I spot the car and pop the trunk. She proceeds to toss the bags in any old way. They land all over the place. Cans are rolling under the spare tire, and I'm in a state of shock. "Do you speak English?" I asked, getting really upset.

"Yes, and very well," she replies.

With no warning, I burst into tears. "Then why won't you talk to me? Didn't they tell you it was part of your job?"

"No," she said. "We don't have to and I'm having a bad day."
Then, I admit, I lost it. "Well, Julia," I say, looking at her name tag, "this may be the last time I ever buy food for my kids who are coming to see me this weekend because I am sick!" I continued, on a rampage now. "Just remember when you are having a bad day, someone else's day may be worse!"

Julia hugs me and says, "I am so very sorry."

Ashamed of myself now, I get in the car and catch a glimpse of my mascara-streaked face. What the hell did you just do, I asked myself.

September 19, 2009
2:30 a.m.

Started the day at the dentist, getting the mouth guard fitted.

Learned all the horrors of no saliva. In addition, my dentist gave me all the gory details of his consultation with my doctors. The more he said "your case," the more panicked I felt.

As soon as I left, I drove over to the radiologist's office. I asked to speak with Dorothy, a very kind nurse. She took me to a private room and turned to give me the biggest hug. It was my medicine. We sat down, and she suggested I buy a chart and make it my "War on Cancer Chart." She explained the visual activity can help patients get through treatment. I do a similar activity with my students, having them use a "dream board" to get through their program and see light at the end of the tunnel. Great idea. Dorothy spent a half hour with me, and it was wonderful to let someone know how that cancer survivor, Jim, scared the crap out of me.

I rushed to Target and got my poster board and new markers. I filled a bag with chemo supplies: new headset, CDs, and reading material. Then I tossed in two new comfortable-type dresses, surprises for Marissa, and a tiara for my granddaughter, Ariana.

My friend Jim invited me to meet him for happy hour at the ocean. He looked handsome, nice haircut, good shoes, decent outfit. I felt pretty and sexy and made a mental note to hang on to that feeling.

* * * * *

Marissa had her first day working at a new spa. She did well. We met at Bonefish for dinner, and I felt so proud of her.

Tomorrow my boys all drive down from Gainesville. Sons George and Ryan and my grandson Evan. Even Jay, my adopted son who is always in his own crisis, is making the effort. I just want to hug each of them and have that connection.

After knowing my friend Jim for ages, I did the craziest thing. I emailed him and for the first time, accepted an invitation for Sinatra and dinner at his house! I just needed to hug and dance slow, one more time in life. Chemo and radiation both start on Monday; I want a good memory to hang on to.

4:00 a.m.

Jim just called me; he can't sleep either! Wow. Great conversation, lots of laughing, and we are on for Sunday night. You mean God gives me cancer, *then* a boyfriend after ten years of just work and kids? This may be my best medicine to kick this thing. There is some joy in my life. Jim told me he is "in" for the duration! I told him that "it's not going to be pretty," and he responded with "I will only say 'poor baby' once or twice, but if I have to kick your butt some days, I will." Isn't he great?

September 19, 2009
Saturday
10:00 a.m.

Cleaning the house and putting clean linens on the beds. My boys are coming today! George, Ryan, Evan, and Jay.

I feel so blessed by God to have this family that loves me. So far, I have received many blessings through this illness, and I am grateful. All I ask for is strength to get through it. Love is everything, and today I feel very loved.

Made my war chart. As cancer is the enemy, I drew mountains to climb and get over to the other side. There are rivers to cross, and all the treatment dates are scattered across the terrain. All these imaginary obstacles along the way correlate with some segment of treatment. At the very end of the chart, I have victory and the last chemo date. I am going to highlight my path, just like Candy Land, grown-up style, more like Stratego.

September 20, 2009
Sunday
6:00 a.m.

Depressed, let down, and wiped out emotionally. Ryan and Jay got drunk and loud and rude. Marissa joined in and wanted to go out to a bar with them. She isn't legal yet, and they didn't need any more. Marissa started crying about "no freedom," and George intervened for me. All hell broke loose, and Ryan and George had words. George said "this isn't about you guys; it's about *our mom sick with cancer,* who needs our support!"

* * * * *

It is now midnight, and I just hid the remaining wine. Then George and Evan sat with me; we had a good talk. George is so let down by his younger brothers. It turned into one of those "when I was fourteen and you forced me to see Dad over summer" conflicts. It was B. S. George kept his cool and repeated "not the right time or place."

There is some jealousy because George has had great success: air force, education, great job, raising two wonderful kids alone. I just can't let their childhood resentments get me down, I need to stay focused on my battle. I know I made mistakes as a parent, but my intentions were always good, always came from a place of love.

After midnight

I made a big meal. Friends Craig and Patricia may stop in; I will save myself emotionally by putting a barrier between me and Ryan and Jay when they call. I saw Evan and George off. He hugged me so tight, and we both broke down.

Now I need to regroup: bubble bath, and nap. Tonight I go over to Jim's, and I want to feel pretty. I have something to look forward to.

Today is the day I decided to live. I am standing up on my own two feet. I thought the four males in my life would make everything better. But they brought their troubles with them. I will rely on me and my God. If TLC (The Learning Channel) was here, the guys could have been in an intervention show. They both abuse alcohol, but I supplied it. I am saving the rest of my strength for the fight of my life, cancer.

My faith has been my cornerstone in life since I was seven years old. When I received my First Holy Communion in the Catholic Church, I literally took Jesus Christ into my heart. Not only do I remember every detail of sitting in the third pew, left side of St. Michael's Church in North Andover, Massachusetts, I remember my conversation and initiation with my Creator. That I know is a gift, to have faith. Years later talking to my siblings, I heard them recall the clothes, the party, the food, and the gifts. I didn't realize until adulthood what a blessing it is to understand, when very young, your place in the universe and never question that, just know.

If you had pain in your childhood, it is okay to feel sorry for yourself—then, own it, just as we must in adulthood, own the life we have and move on.

September 21, 2009
Monday
4:00 a.m.

Chemotherapy and radiation day! Wow, just writing that hurts. My prayer is to be able to endure and have nothing be unbearable. That is all I can ask God. The boys left early yesterday morning. I got to share a bowl of cereal with Evan alone, while the house was quiet. These are the gifts of life. My tall, sweet, handsome grandson just talking with me about life. His wisdom at sixteen, so inspiring.

George was all business until he hugged me bye. I will never forget being enveloped by my son's strong arms. My baby when I was just nineteen, now an ironic turn of life, our roles reversed.

Whatever George's one-on-one with Marissa was, it seemed to take, and Marissa turned the corner into kindness.

Ryan had been in tears and shambles, asking if he could stay to help me get through this. Through our tears I had to say no, knowing that he has his own demons to fight before he can help me.

Jay was cold, and it hurts. When you adopt a child at age seven from the foster-care system, part of them loves you, and the other part resents you. You are not the biological parent who pulled it together and retrieved them. His arrogance is his emotional shield, and I get it. Nonetheless, ouch! Someday he will get it and realize he has a family and safe place to land. Eleven more years in the system, until eighteen, would have injured his spirit even more.

My brunch with pals Dr. Craig and Patricia was what I needed before today. Craig shared he had been struggling with his own medical situation and hid it from me. Now with growing enemies in our bodies, we bonded closer.

* * * * *

My expectations were too high about my date with Jim. After all the "works"—perfume, make-up, and hair—I entered his house to beautiful music, candles, and cocktails. Emotionally depleted from my weekend, as soon as he got on my nerves, I bolted. I guess it was "fight or flight." On my drive home, I had to laugh at myself for thinking I could put "emotional fulfillment" on my appointment book and be able to check it off.

Then I cried. A call to my friend Robert lifted me up enough to get me over the hump. When I came home, Rissy's nurturing arms were finally there.

10:30 a.m.

Now I'm sitting in the chemo chair shivering under three blankets. They just put the third bag of solution in my IV. How stupid was I to buy a new dress for chemotherapy! Note to self—next time, warm sweats and socks.

Terry the nurse is sweet and very funny. How would you be able to cope with all this pain daily, without a good sense of humor? Marissa and DeeAnn went out to breakfast after dropping me off; I could see the fear in their eyes and played it cool. Now it feels like I'm sitting on a block of ice naked. The man in the recliner next to me looks dead. One day down, two months to go.

By noon time, I have eaten all my snacks, read all my magazines, and listened to my new CDs. Now I watch and listen as people beg for more pain killers and argue with the nurses. Six hours drag on.

This is a living hell! Bright fluorescent lights, human skeletons making their way to the bathrooms, dragging their IV poles. People vomiting or crying, horrid smells and that TV Dr. Feinstein bragged about flickers on and off with Kathie Lee and Hoda.

I tried to lend my *Architectural Digest* to the lady on the other side of me, but it was too heavy for her and hit the floor. Neither of us could pick it up with all our tubes hooked up. I watched a port being changed on a child. I thought about how at this time on a Monday I'm usually in my air-conditioned office, looking out at the palm trees when I take a break from my work. I have been very sheltered. I pray this works.

September 22, 2009
Tuesday
8:00 a.m.

What a beautiful, sunny day. I awoke with no pain. I made some coffee. Patricia spent the night; she's still asleep. Donna called to check on me. All is well. Radiation last night was rough. There was a two and a half hour delay, so I had time to get myself in a nervous frenzy. Gina and Rissy both were with me for support. Everyone came in calm. Not as traumatic as chemo. Just when I was calming down, they called me in. My head was literally snapped to the table by a Hannibal Lector mask. They stuck a wax spoon in my mouth like I was having shock therapy. They did not want me to bite my tongue. Away I went into the tunnel. The movie *Snake Pit* popped into my mind. I had to remind myself that this is the cure, not the punishment. Six acts of contrition and two rosaries later, it finally stopped. I came out woozy, and the girls lovingly helped me.

Up since 4:00 a.m., I was wiped out. When we got to the house, two dear girlfriends, Blanca and Jahira were waiting for me with their kids. Just when I watered down the soup, Patricia showed up with her overnight bag. Dinner for seven!

Just put my PJs on and checked my email. Jim called to say he was always there if I needed him and good luck with treatment.

I highlighted the first ring on my cancer chart. I asked God to bless all the loving hands of the medical staff who saw me through.

3:30

Put a very healthy dinner on to cook, had a nap, ate some broth. Catching up on emails from loved ones. George's said, "Mom, if there was a way I could take the suffering for you, I would. I love you so very much. Mom, we all need you and I love you. I'm full of gratitude for all you have done for me and my siblings." Wiped me out on that one.

My dear friend Robert called, such a good guy, cards are arriving daily, lovely Debra McDonald left all her numbers for me. She's in social services, so it means a lot.

Still trying to refinance my house. My neighbor Shannon just came by to see if I needed anything; people are good.

September 22, 2009
9:00 p.m.

Drive myself to Radiology *alone*. I don't know what happened to me, but when they took the helmet off me, I started crying. Cancer has made me so vulnerable. When I came home to an empty house, I had a big bowl of ice cream, like a little kid rewarding herself.

Gina called. "Yes," I answered to the question she asked after I told her my situation. "I will spend tomorrow night over there." Sounds better than this pity party I'm having with chunky monkey.

September 23, 2009
7:00 a.m.

I kept swatting the alarm button until I realized the sound was from the phone. My sister Donna, walking her dog up North in the cool fall air, was checking in. I, on the other hand, awoke in a mass of sweat, my nightgown was tangled and I felt like I had had my first glass of razor blades. Just like the "cancer supporter" warned me so graciously. I took a spoonful of pain killer for the first time and tried to get it past what felt like beach sand stuck in my throat. Thank God it kicked in and now I get it. The special tooth paste, mouth gel, the whole shebang. I'm going to go back to sleep before the meds wear off.

10:30 a.m.

Marissa just woke me before she went to work. This is a record for me. I'm wiped out. The dietician left a message on my phone: "are you getting enough calories?" I dragged myself to the kitchen and made a Boost shake with coffee. Set it up, pushed the button, and everything flowed all over the place. The seal broke on the bottom of the blender. (Well, it sat in a box for twenty years.)

Then I tried my old food processor. This time I threw in coffee, Boost, and a banana. Hit the blend button. Silence. Next, I poured the concoction into a bowl and used my mom's hand mixer from 1961. Bingo! On payday, I'll splurge for a new blender. As the sticky liquid continued to run down the cupboards, I realized I was exhausted from just breakfast.

Just when I got things cleaned up and was going to lay back down, my daughter Rachel called. I adopted her at ten years old, and in some ways she is emotionally stuck in childhood. She gabs about her neighbors, her in-laws, and just about anything I don't care about. I can barely hang on and listen, but I know she means well. Soon I had to yell "gotta go!" because the shake was returning.

September 24, 2009
7:00 a.m.

Sitting in my granddaughter Ariana's pink princess bedroom. I spent the night after radiation. What a safe feeling to be in a child's room. She has butterfly curtains, a big doll house, and pink linens. Just for a night I could forget I'm the mom, the parent who pays the bills. I'm still nauseous, but I'm going to make the three grandkids a big breakfast and then do an art project with them. It feels so safe to be here with Gina's family. For so many years, she was one of those "critical daughters" who thought I did not do anything right. Since my diagnosis, she's grown up and been so loving and helpful. What a blessing.

By the time I drove home, I was a dish rag. Collapsing on the sofa, I passed out. Next thing I know, two ladies I haven't seen in years show up. No call, no invitation. What is with people? They came to satisfy their curiosity, and I was annoyed. To be the freak people come to view, is how I felt. Today I'm the baby with the third arm.

Night Time, Same Day

Hey, I'm feeling good. I am so grateful and thrilled to not be sick. DeeAnn drove me to tonight's radiation, and Marissa had dinner waiting when we returned, Alfredo with pasta. The laundry was all folded! Feeling so much better, I phoned George to share it. My son's genuine happiness for me made my night. Marissa is being sweeter, my friend DeeAnn was supportive, and George wished me a good night. Just for this moment, life is good: no pain, no nausea. I drifted off to sleep with a sense of peace. Hooray!

September 25, 2009
Friday
3:30 a.m.

Just got sick to my stomach, totally disgusting. This is when I'm glad *not* to have a partner beside me. Okay, what did I learn?

1. Do not skip the anti-nausea medicine!
2. Don't eat salad or roughage!
3. Have water and gum or mints on the nightstand (for after clean-up).
4. Leave the bedroom door open. It is a straight run to the guest bath; the master bath has two doors to maneuver.

* * * * *

Life is flying by me. I feel like crap today, but I need to go in to work. It took me until 11:30 a.m. to pull it together. When I walked into the break room, everyone stopped talking. Everyone looked up at me as if I were the walking dead. It's funny: I hadn't noticed the physical changes in me yet.

Oh, it feels good to put my key in my office door! Still fits. Went over some lesson plans with the substitute and wore myself out.

Tonight, Radiation Number Five

I had no one to go with, feeling very alone. After a long day, I dragged myself in. Marissa was starting dinner. As we finished up together, we were deathly quiet, just really sad. "Why don't you get the mail while I set the table," I said solemnly.

Wow! Marissa returned with a giant box from my sister Donna. All kinds of goodies: old photos, new CDs, various hats, Jell-o, and even a small white board (lap size) with markers for when I lose my voice. There was also a card from my other sister, Pat, with $100.00 in it! Perfect timing. These gifts got us out of our funk and into a better mood. Suddenly we were laughing and talking.

Bedtime

Now I dread sleep. It is horrible to wake up and do the bathroom run, sick as a dog. It is lonely to lock up the house and go upstairs alone. I haven't heard from David yet, not one call, though we were married almost eighteen years. Still hurts.

September 27, 2009
Sunday
1:00 p.m.

What a blessing the weekends, with the break from treatments, are and also, this weekend, Craig is driving up from Miami to take me to lunch.

Last night, I read Lance Armstrong's book, and it helped me cope.

Still working on my battle chart; now I look forward to the climb. Took all my get-well cards and made a collage. New music from Donna is playing, and I left a message for the carpet cleaner. Life goes on. People get sick and carpets get dirty.

9:30 p.m.

Heard from my dear friend Maria; she is a gift from God. She and her husband, Paul, have been so very supportive. He is in the medical field and has many resources they offered so generously. We have a meeting on campus this week to see if I can get her approved as my sub in the future, if I need more time.

Today I had fun with Craig at lunch. He showed up in a brand-new, silver, two-seater Mercedes. He looked great in a tank top and bermudas. We are so compatible; too bad he's gay: I just love him!

Well, he took me to an upscale place on the water. We sat out on the deck and were having good conversation. All of a sudden, the snooty manager comes over and says, "Sir, do you have a shirt in your car?" He did not, so we had a hasty lunch and left.

I was so upset that when I got home, I posted a crappy review online and signed it.

Marissa went out on a date with a new boy tonight. I pray she is safe.

Tomorrow big day—chemo very early.

September 28, 2009
Monday
5:30 a.m.

"Good morning, Lord. Offering us a New Day, untouched and freshly new, and here I am to ask you, Lord, if you'll renew me, too. Forgive me for the errors I made yesterday, and help me walk closer to thy way."

For twelve years, Marissa and I recited those words in the car on the way to school. This morning they came back so clearly.

Do I dread my chemo today? No. Do I look forward to it? No. I believe God chose me for this challenge, chose me to learn some valuable lessons. Yes, I accept what has been assigned to me.
My clarity and humanity are right there for me. I have never been a multi-tasking, automatic-pilot person. I know each moment is part of a divine script. Who the heck am I to do rewrites? So I pack my chemo bag as I would my brief case or school backpack. I show up on time and even with a smile. All the while I know I am experiencing life to the fullest. Nothing gets past me. Just observing people's eyes and body language tells me so much.

There's a woman in the radiologist's office who deposits her husband's wheelchair in the waiting room. She never touches his shoulder or says a word. It hurts me to watch them. She goes out front to sit on a bench with her book. His pale eyes reveal that he had given up as a man.

The tone of the nurses' voices tells the patients "you are a pain in the ass" or "I value you as a worthwhile human being." Luckily for me so far, I have been treated with dignity. My eyes are wide open, and I'm not wading through cancer.

I can experience every bit with acceptance and then interpret my creator's message to me.

September 29, 2009
Tuesday
2:00 a.m.

I am visualizing rotisserie chickens, with the long metal rods going through them from side to side. My head is going round and round in the glass case in the deli. My earaches are hot pockets searing through my skull. My headache pressure is building, as if it is about to uncork. I don't want to vomit—I hate it—so I rummage through the pill basket and find two extra-strength Tylenol. Sipping a Sprite, I realize this is my new addiction. Just enough carbonation and ice cold; I can keep it down!

A little TV and I try to sleep. Pound, pound, pound. No way. Now I'm in the garage in my nightgown, shivering, trying to find some Coke. No luck. Just an empty carton.

* * * * *

Why wouldn't Marissa be selfish? For eighteen years, I put her first; I created the monster.

Note to self—move the tiny fridge to my room and keep it stocked for myself. Mom needs help!

In a way, I am glad that Donna left before she had to see me suffer and that Marissa is saving herself emotionally.

As soon as I get paid, I'll pick up my pain-killer prescription. That's it in a nutshell: it costs money to have cancer!

Losing track of time without the routine of work. My only job now is to get well.

Last night was hell. Rissy and I had Chinese food. Big mistake, let's not even go there. After two grueling hours, mercifully, I dozed off. I awoke to a fireball in my throat. I hope it means the tumor is breaking up from treatment.

Putting the TV on to distract myself from the pain, a boring show on stocks and bonds was on. A line jumped out at me: "know when to enter and when to exit." Simple, yet brilliant. I started to think about jobs, relationships, and every other area of life that requires timing.

Too bad we aren't given this advice as kids. We would save ourselves a lot of heartache. Thinking of the times I should have pushed myself to try something new or stick to a difficult task. Never mind relationships or jobs when I stayed too long at the fair.

Unfortunately, it takes so many years and so many hurts to get to this point. If I make it to the other side of cancer, I hope to remember this. And also to be a little kinder to everyone.

6:00 a.m.

Marissa came home all chirpy and cheerful. She brought me cold water, very sweet, but I shut the lights out at 5:15 a.m. Now she had a tray of dry toast for me. Rather than rock the boat, I try to get it down, past the fireball. Next, she lit her sage incense and the whole house smells like hippie armpits. Closing my eyes and blocking my nose helps. Then Marissa yells from the kitchen: "Mom, how does onions, peppers, and mushrooms sound for my omelette?" Gotta love her. Clueless.

Afternoon

My face is green. My eyes are sunk in my head. I stare at myself in the mirror: "who is that?" I can no longer breathe easily, and I smear Vicks on my face, neck, and head. It helps, and the soothing smell reminds me of my loving mom when I was little. It takes every ounce of energy I have left to drag myself to the shower. I start to lose my balance and have to sit on the shower floor.

When I finish, I collapse on my bed. Here comes Marissa in her bikini; she's carrying her beach bag. It is actually a relief to know the house will be quiet again. As I drift off, I pray: God, please don't let her drown.

Bedtime, 9:00 p.m.

After a day of feeling like scum on the bottom of a fish-bait bucket, I dragged my butt to radiation. My friend Robert called and was so kind and sweet. I cried all the way into the building. My emotions are so raw. Robert offered to sit with me in chemo on Monday. He lost a love to cancer years ago; that devastated him. It means so much to me that he is willing to put himself out there once again.

Tonight Dr. Bushbaum is not here. His young "fill-in" introduces himself. He scans my chart and weighs me in, down five more pounds. Something in me knew he was new at this, so without hesitating, I said, "Doctor, would you refresh my memory? What stage cancer did Dr. Bushbaum tell me I was in?"

As he flips through the chart, he cheerfully says "here it is! Stage four A."

I almost fainted. For some reason I was thinking stage two or three, at the most. I did not want to show any emotion so he would not know he had spilled the beans. Walking into the treatment room, I said to myself, "You want to play with the big boys, you gotta take it." Just keep your cool; keep on moving.

After treatment I sat in my car. I kept saying "stage four" to myself. What does "A" mean? Is "B" death? I called Marissa, and she met me at Dunkin' Donuts. She was too shut down for me to turn to. Here I am, again, alone with the cat and a newspaper. Marissa went out with friends.

It is not only the suffering that frightens me; I am not ready to leave my loved ones. God help me!

September 30, 2009
4:00 a.m.

Awakening with tears streaming down my face. My subconscious is preparing me to leave this earth. Is this my transitional phase into eternal life? Will I only watch in spirit form Marissa and Kendra's weddings? I am in a state of shock. Of course, I knew I was very sick, but stage four? The expression "don't buy any ripe bananas" kept popping into my brain.

3:00 p.m.

Marissa and I had a doozy of a fight. Crying, yelling, and, finally, comforting each other by hugging. We are in so much emotional pain.

Reaching a truce, I sent Marissa to do errands with my ATM card. I do worry if she is responsible enough, but I'm sick as a bloody dog. Everything now tastes like metal chips, and I alternate between not being able to go to the bathroom and just making it in time. My body betrayed me! Now I need two or three naps a day. I am not sure, honestly, that I will make it.

October 1, 2009

Back at my married daughter, Gina's, house. Just played two games of Concentration with three freshly scrubbed grandkids. Lots of laughter, ice cream, and hugs. There were a few pouts over losing, but this is the stuff life is made of. I have wasted precious time. Too much time has been spent on career and not enough on family. Since I found out my cancer was advanced, I am clinging to life. I am in love with everyone. I want to curl up in a ball with each loved one and fall asleep in their arms. I feel so vulnerable.

Last night, I slept at a girlfriend's house. Six women surrounded me to give me a healing treatment as I was on the floor, covered by a large towel. My dear friend Ann Marie arranged it, and it took place at her home. Everyone was in some "healing modality": esthetics, massage, nursing, and reflexology. Ann Marie sent her daughter to go get Marissa to join us. Thrilled to see her walk through the door, I didn't care if she had a cocktail with Ann Marie's daughter. Marissa needed the healing as much as I did. I am so impressed by these women. Surrounded by life and love!

Beautiful music played, everyone helped with the meal, and Ann Marie took out her best china and crystal.

I am so grateful for dear friends. Today, I missed a Cancer Alliance meeting in Delray, but it was worth it for the beautiful gift of life I received.

I tiptoed out of Ann Marie's at sunrise, leaving a love note of thanks. They gave me hope!

Then a successful meeting at the college to go over the 2010 schedule. My dear friend Maria got the job to be my "permanent" substitute. Everyone went to lunch together. I pretended to eat soup, but nothing is getting past the scar tissue now. That's okay; it felt wonderful to be part of the working world.

After my radiation treatment, I drove out to work and Gina's house. Just love this family neighborhood: kids on bikes, neighbors watering lawns, everyone waves hello. Just how I grew up. (My townhouse is smack in the middle of my building, and it feels very isolated to me.)

My son-in-law Mark, the pastor, has a pool service to help support his family. Gina and Mark were at the dining-room table doing his billing together. I jumped in and sealed and stamped invoices. What a thrill to be alive and part of a family business, if only for an hour.

In twenty-four hours, I have taken part in at least a dozen people's rich lives. Part of my loneliness, I see now, was my selfishness in remaining aloof. Without the cancer, I would still be in my bubble.

October 2, 2009
Friday
10:00 p.m.

Sitting here in the dark. A fuse blew out. I am writing by the light from a fifteen-watt battery-operated night light. Today I hit bottom again. Rushing home from Gina's to meet the carpet cleaners, I discovered Marissa had not moved a thing and was not prepared for the workers to begin. She wasn't home so I frantically moved everything by myself.

My whole body feels as though I ran a marathon. Lifting a pencil hurts. I placed my Rubbermaid stool in the shower, as I can no longer stand for the length of time the shower takes. Mouth sores have erupted, and I cannot swallow past the throat tumors now. Every thing makes me sick now, even a diaper commercial.

After the carpet cleaners left, I laid down. Marissa came in and said "what's for dinner?" like a demanding husband. All I could muster was "you're a big girl and I can't even swallow water now. Figure it out." Back and forth until we both broke down in tears. I threw my water glass across the room, and it broke in a million pieces on the tile floor. Then I sat in the shower and sobbed my eyes out.

When I drove myself to radiation and got into the office, a nice woman took one look at my face and took both my hands in hers. "Carol" was so kind. That was all I needed. We sat quietly together, waiting for our turns.

When I left radiation, I knew my body needed nourishment. Managing to keep a scrambled egg down at Denny's was a victory. I then picked up the "magic" mouthwash supplies at the pharmacy. They are supposed to numb and disinfect at once.

Now sitting here in the dark, I feel helpless. I phoned Marissa, and she was out to eat with friends. When I told her about the electricity being out, she said, "Mom, just go in the garage and flip the switches." There is no way I am going into a pitch-black garage to fool around with electricity tonight. What is God trying to teach me? Is it that I need people?

Donna arrives in two days to help me. It takes me twice as long to do one simple chore as it used to, so I am ready for some help. Thankfully, I have two days off treatment to try and prepare the house. I will try my hardest to get out of this funk and focus on the positive! Here's the short list:

1. Picked up new nausea and pain meds
2. Donna is coming!
3. Still on the payroll
4. New book to read (in the event the lights come back on)

Think! Where is there a flashlight? I'm being a baby, but I don't want to step in a puddle and get shocked. Just call it a night, I tell myself. The sun will come out tomorrow. (Okay, Annie.)

October 3, 2009
10:00 a.m.

Last night I awoke and could not make it further than the sink to be sick. Actually wet myself at the same time. So much for the new meds!

Towels, clothes, rugs—what a mess! I just rolled it up until morning. Now, if I felt better it would be worth it, but no. This went on all night. When the sun came up, I, in my nightgown, was in the driveway, hosing off rugs.

* * * * *

Crazy thoughts race through my head, can't die unless the house is clean. It takes me forty minutes on my knees to put clean sheets on the bed for Donna's visit. Everything that cancer survivor told me is true. Still, I would have found out on my own. Even water hurts me now, and it tastes like cat food. I'm getting thinner and weaker.

Who could ever stand me like this except my Creator? At 5:00 a.m. I pull out my dusty Bible. As usual, I open to the words I need at this moment:

> To have faith is to be sure of things we cannot see. It was by their faith that God's People of ancient times won God's approval.
>
> It is by faith that we understand the universe was created by God's *word*, so that what can be *seen* was made of what cannot be seen. (Hebrews 11: 1-3)

3:00 p.m.

Just took a Valium, jumping out of my skin. Trying to brainstorm. How do I get through five more weeks of hell?

Just read in the morning paper about the lunatic who kidnapped and raped Elizabeth Smart. That girl kept her wits about her, every single day of torture! Surely I can do this chemo thing. When I stop to think of our prisoners of war over the years, like John McCain, to have broken bones, unattended, locked in dark boxes. What is the common thread that enables people to endure? Faith. Even Jesus said from the cross, "Father, why have you forsaken me?" Surely a wimp like me can endure a little longer.

Marissa came home with groceries. Hallelujah!

Bedtime 9:30 p.m.

Made it through one more day. Gave myself a bubble bath and had a cold ginger ale with a Benedryl to knock myself out. I have not been able to use the bathroom, so I drank mineral oil straight from the bottle. Hopefully, in the morning it does the trick.

Online, I did some research on George's hospital—Shands Hospital at the University of Florida. They have a well-known cancer center. Sending George an email asking if my treatment does not work how he would feel about me going up there. I do not want to intrude on his life.

I miss the old days when sick people could stay in the hospital and get back rubs and cold pitchers of water. The nurses were like a buzzer away. Now I'm up and down three flights of stairs in my townhouse. Just worn out and trying to hang on.

Marissa had a family event at Nick's. I hope it gets her mind off cancer, and she has a break.

October 4, 2009
Sunday morning

The pain got more severe during the night. I lost the ability to swallow any pills. Even the liquid meds are getting impossible. Then I discovered an old box of popsicles in the freezer. They saved me. Now I'll rest.

October 5, 2009
2:30 p.m.

Finished my third round of chemotherapy. Enya CD *And The Winter Came* from Maria and Paul on my headset got me through it. When I opened my eyes, there were Donna and Rissy together, their blue eyes sparkling. They wore vivid green and pink. Together they were a magnificent sight. What a gift to have loved ones that care for me.

October 6, 2009
Tuesday

Busy, busy, very sick day. Donna helped me get a lot accomplished, but I overdid it and my body gave out. Today would have been my thirty-fifth anniversary with Dave. Still no word. In bed by 8:00 p.m. Sad.

October 7, 2009
Wednesday

Donna rushed me to the oncologist today. They put me on a special IV to get my hydration up. The blood work concerned Dr. Feinstein, and he gave me a night off radiation. Out of it. Thank God my sister is here.

October 8, 2009

Pain, pain, and more pain. Having a teaspoon of Roxy, a painkiller, every four hours. My ears are burned from the radiation; it's as if a drill is going through my skull. Nightmare about David and me trying to protect the kids, all terror and upsetting, nothing good. Still working on my war chart, when I can.

October 10, 2009
Saturday night

Lost a day somehow. Tried to force a banana smoothie down, cannot even get water past the neck lumps now. The earaches are the worst.

Donna had to leave, so very sad. My girlfriend Terry Kawalic came to drive me to radiation. I can no longer drive, or I shouldn't. All over her beautiful Camry, I got sick. She pulled over on the side of the highway, and I rolled in the grass on the side of the road. Terry helped me out of my clothes and wrapped me in a beach towel from her trunk. She had a roll of paper towels and plastic bags, even a gallon of water she used to rinse me off. One more attack, repeat performance, before we made it home. How in the world do people make themselves throw up on purpose? It is the most horrid experience.

My hair is starting to fall out. DeeAnn lent me a wig, and I tried it on. I did some make-up and looked in the mirror. It was 1975, and I was Carol Brady. I have lost all objectivity.

Cancer sucks. My life is forever changed. Piles of hair are on my pillow.

My bills are piling up, too. At night, I'm dreaming about Thanksgiving dinner. What a blessing to be able to eat delicious food. Being healthy is such a gift from God. The ability to work, eat, live. Wow! If or when I get through this, I will enjoy my life forever. I will go to dinner more. Maybe have a man in my life, maybe even a husband!

I love the routine of holidays and birthdays, even washing clothes. When was the last time I held a newborn baby or handed out Halloween candy? I want to be able to decorate another Christmas tree, dance, eat, travel, and work. Note to self: do not isolate!

Enjoy life's little pleasures every single day. Reach out to others and help anyone I possibly can.

Still having painful dreams about David. Lots of work, still, to do on myself. The cancer made me face the painful things I buried.

October 11, 2009
Sunday
10:00 a.m.

Slept thirteen hours straight. Feeling almost human. The weight is still dropping, and I'm looking rundown. Today I am going to do some chores. Doctor Craig is coming to see me! I am managing an iced coffee with a *Sopranos* rerun on. For a little bit, life almost feels normal. I'll worry about my chemo tomorrow. (Okay, Scarlet.)

Next on the agenda—start planning a life after cancer. I want a partner and a home. This solitary life is not as great as I thought it would be. I thought I wanted to be like Henry David Thoreau. I changed my mind.

October 12, 2009
Monday
4:15 p.m.

There is a line in the movie *Bucket List* where Morgan Freeman says to Jack Nicholson, "never trust a fart." Cute line, now totally hysterical, so side-splitting funny I can't catch my breath. No more needs to be said on that.

Marissa dropped me, three bags, and a cooler off at chemotherapy. I dragged myself in for vital signs. Not good. I know bedside chat is not Dr. Feinstein's thing, but he tried. Very dehydrated, three collapsed veins, lost another four pounds, but blood work is not that bad. Verdict: chemo must go on.

Finally, they find a vein. I get the extra IV today, to build me up. Larry from work came by to see me, means so much to me. Nice shirt and tie. Catching up on work news. Then my dear co-worker and friend Heidi popped in. She reminds me of the old Kathleen, living and loving her married life and children. Oh, to be able to turn back the clock. I find myself asking her what she is cooking for dinner, just to relive those memories, school projects, church activities: all the good stuff. A shared life.

When Marissa came to pick me up, she was still cranky. She a slow burn, and I'm a hit and run. I regret my temper as soon as I lose it. Terry the nurse tried to warm Marissa up, but she was not having it.

I am daydreaming about cashing in my retirement and just opting out of life. I could just say screw it and enjoy what time I have left. Now I get it, why people just give up and leave everything and everyone behind.

October 15, 2009
Hospital, day two

I was hospitalized and had surgery today. The feeding tube is in. Tomorrow I will have a lesson in usage. Lots has transpired since I last wrote. I ended up driving myself to radiation. It was one of the worst I ever had. It all blew up in one quick night. When I got off the radiation table, I felt they [had given] me an extra dose. I was very shaky and disoriented. The tech was trying to put me at ease, but the thought of those beams so close to my spinal column scared the hell out of me.

As I was leaving, Gina and the kids pulled up in the parking lot to see me. It was so very thoughtful, but I was wiped out. It was double-whammy day, six hours of chemo and then radiation at night. We had a hot, short visit in Gina's van. By the time I was behind the wheel, I was deathly ill.

Then I got lost. (This I can do even when I am not sick.) Driving in circles, sweating, and trying not to go off the road, I found some old tissues to be sick in. Now I'm crying and nothing looks familiar. I called Rissy on the cell. "Mom! Look out the window," she said. "Read me the signs!" She was exasperated with me. Nothing rang a bell; I knew I was not even coherent at this point.

Then it dawns on me. I am dehydrated from no liquids, and I am having some post-traumatic symptoms from treatment. I pulled into the first parking lot I could find and get out of the car. There is no sign on the building I walk up to, but there is a big doorbell and intercom grate. I press the bell.

"South Florida Mental Health of Delray. How can we help you?" Oh, my God, I am even in the wrong city. An attendant in a white jacket opens the door. I was crying so hard it took a minute for him to realize I was not there to be admitted. He calmly gave me directions home and some free therapy. He told me his mom had head and neck cancer back in 1984. "How did she make out?" I asked.

"She passed away three weeks ago at age ninety-three. She never relapsed."

Well, either he is a great liar or God sent me to this place to hear something hopeful. She had twenty-five more years of life! I left with directions, totally calmed down.

It was a rough night of alternating between having the shakes under six quilts or cranking up the heating pad. All night freeze, vomit, shakes, then fry. The little bit I know about medicine made me think my body was going into shock. Finally, daylight came, and I phoned the oncologist. He said to meet him right away at the hospital, and four days later I am coming out of it and have a tube dangling from my abdomen.

When I first came to, I saw David. Then all my kids and my niece, who flew in from Virginia. From everyone's faces, I knew it was a close call.

October 19, 2009

Crying, sobbing, and vomiting, I hit the wall in the hospital. They sent in an Indian psychiatrist to see me. The first thing he said was "why a pretty lady like you divorced?"

I tried to explain that I had stage-four cancer and the divorce was many years ago.

"No wonder so sad. We talk about why no husband."

This was beyond weird; then I remembered my Indian students telling me about their arranged marriages and how their families considered divorce to be like death. I had to regroup and play along to get something to help me out.

After I gave him enough weepy divorce details, he ordered an antidepressant for me. Never have I believed in them! Never say never.

They also put a morphine patch on me that takes the edge off.

When I was released, they forgot to give me any tube formula. Now my weight is going very low, and within two days I was back at Dr. Feinstein's getting that special IV again. I have a case of shingles, stress-related and chronic.

Marissa blew the family budget while I was in the hospital. She kept all the out-of-town guests fed well.

Ryan came and stayed. Emotionally, he is a help, but financially, he is another person to care for.

My radiation is back on daily; I'm working my war chart and trying to hang in a few more weeks. I was at the devil's door, and I was spared.

October 22, 2009
7:00 a.m.

Dave visited me two more times! I feel good about it, but I hate that look on his face! I remember when we were first married he wrote me a letter that said "your beauty scares me." Well, now I'm scaring him in the opposite way. Cancer really sucks. It smells, it hurts, and it takes away your core. I pray to lick this thing and *live* again.

2:00 p.m.

Feeling better! I am thrilled to hold a little something down. Today I rested. Radiation called; all the computers are down. No treatment tonight. Shocked. I was actually disappointed. This throws off my war chart, and I can see the finish line. Now between the hospitalization and the broken radiology computers, I'm falling way behind. The cancellation came so late DeeAnn was already on her way over. She insisted on us driving out there anyway to pick up my new formula prescription. Nice to have a little break with my friend.

When I returned home, Ryan helped me with the feeding tube. I was so proud of him. (Rissy ran for the hills.) What a reversal of roles; my six-foot-tall son feeding me formula. I'm feeling so vulnerable, and when Ryan leaves this time, I will miss him.

October 24, 2009

The pain is under control! How wonderful is that. Even though I still feel like the walking dead. Each foot is a lead weight; however, the pain patch blurs the acuteness of the throat pain.

The visiting nurses are coming today. I am depending on them. I am only having nourishment once a day, and only if someone helps me. Ryan left, and Marissa is too squeamish to try. DeeAnn helped me yesterday. My arms are not long enough to do it alone; if there is not enough gravity, the flow stops. It actually takes three hands to do it right. Infection scares the hell out of me. Then I get mad at myself for being a wimp.

Last night Patricia cancelled my radiation at the last minute; she said she had a fever. Right before she called, Dave had called to ask if I need "anything at all." So I took him up on it after Patricia cancelled, and I called him back for a ride. So Dave took me to treatment. Can life get any stranger? It felt like we came full circle back to friendship.

* * * * *

Now I'm on my bed in a ball, just waiting for some help. If none arrives, I will bite the bullet and just take care of myself to stay alive.

Later

After I had waited six hours, the nurse showed up. She showed me a different method to using the feeding tube. I am more relaxed about it now; I guess there is more than one way to skin a cat.

October 26, 2009

Happy Birthday to me. Yesterday I turned sixty! That hurt to even write down. Who would believe I would not be able to enjoy a birthday meal? Sick as a dog. Cancer is hell. I pray if I don't get to remission, God takes me fast.

Marissa is still shut down. Craig sent flowers and so did Gina and Mark. Craig brought his new puppy over; it gave me a lift.

* * * * *

After I fell asleep, I woke up abruptly, covered in vomit. My bedroom smells of death, even with the carpet cleaned. I sweat toxins out, from the chemo, constantly.

Marissa planned on driving me to chemo, but it is hard to get her up on time. Very little fight left, and I need to step it up to *Live*! So many people just roll over: where do others get their courage? My faith is still strong, but on bad days I ask myself does it matter what side of life I'm on? Eternal spiritual life or the agony of the physical life here on Earth.

October 30, 2009
Friday
4:00 a.m.

Burning in pain. My ears are two hot coals. My throat is raw. I now cannot make it to the bathroom to be sick. My nice clean bed is destroyed over and over. I phone Marissa downstairs and just mutter "emergency."

I haven't written the last few days because the suffering has been too much. My rib cage aches like knives are thrust in it. Yesterday, I drove myself to the oncologist for a special IV treatment. I lost two and a half more pounds. Once again we changed the formula; none of them agree with me. New one? Even worse. Everything comes right back up. So beaten down.

When Terry the chemo nurse saw me, she put her hand on the arm of the chair, slid it to the edge and said, "This is you. The chair is death. Just when you are about to go over the edge, we snatch you back!" With that, she dramatically pulls her fingers back. My question is how do they know when to snatch you back?

My house is full of cards and flowers. However, it could be a new car. Nothing matters. I am going to need more incentive to live. So far, nothing has given me a reason.

I spend another night at Gina and Mark's. At breakfast, she told me that last night we had had a two-hour talk about life. Every pain we ever endured or gave each other, we got out. She said we both cried our eyes out. I have no recollection of any of it! How strange is that? The meds are working.

In forty-eight hours, Donna will be here. I feel desperate for help and care. Just when I felt like giving up, my friend (a massage therapist) showed up. Cristene rubbed her magic oils on my feet with love and tenderness.

7:30 a.m.

The Motrin helped my ears. The pain is bearable. I awake drenched in sweat, very disoriented. I heard from the bank. I'm late on my payments. Cancer is so expensive. Even with major medical, I owe thousands. There are seven or eight new prescriptions per week. The last antibiotic was $65.00, so I left it at the pharmacy. The oncologist said I am very susceptible to picking something up due to my compromised immune system.

Later

DeeAnn called Donna in Boston to say I am getting worse and that she has to fly to Chicago with her husband. Donna heard her and extended her visit. How loving was that?

If I ever needed my family, it's now. I pray for God's mercy. In the morning I open my eyes and dread each waking moment.

I have a high pain tolerance. I have had two ten-pound babies, a dozen gallstones, and surgery. All kinds of weird close calls medically, but cancer takes the cake.

October 31, 2009
Halloween

Always hated Halloween. Gory, stupid holiday about frightening kids. Being disrespectful to the dead and, lately, it has become like a religion.

Commercials, candy, costumes, every talk show is about how to throw a party and make the food look like brains on a plate. Whatever happened to hay rides and bobbing for apples?

Just woke up in pain. My back went out when I made up the guest bed for Donna. Every day, Marissa says, "tomorrow I'll do it." Finally, only twenty-four hours left; I just did it. Now this pulled muscle is going in spasms. Complaint department closed. The self-pity is the worst of it; I have to fight the negativity. I just want to know if I will live or die. Will I keep a roof over our heads? What does the future hold?

12:30 a.m.

Wake up to check on Marissa. She went to a Halloween party, and her bed is empty. So I called her cell; she sounds tipsy. Great, I'm laid up and she's pushing the limits. She said she is staying at a friend's tonight. What can I do? I would rather she stay put than drink and drive.

I'm exceptionally thirsty. I can only take baby sips of water, so I used the stomach peg for just liquid. I'm almost glad I have no partner to witness this odd procedure.

I called Geo today and cried. Hated to dump my problems on one of my kids, but I'm against the wall.

Gina came over with the kids. I paid them twenty-five cents a bag of laundry if they hauled it to their van. Gina's helping me keep it up. The rest of the chores, I paid for with cookies. Gina was kind to me and gave me a shoulder rub. How sad it took all these years for my oldest girl to touch me lovingly.

Precious sleep comes over me.

Tomorrow my dear sister returns.

November 2, 2009
Sunday!

Long, long day of waiting for Donna. We turned the clocks back, so it is even longer. Feeling slightly better. Prayers are being answered. This restlessness is maddening! I'm jumping out of my skin. Rissy is picking up Donna for me; they should be here by 9:00 p.m. God, just keep all of us safe until we meet up later tonight. I'm hanging on!

My son-in-law Mark came by to fix my broken washer. No luck. Nothing is easy.

November 11, 2009

Haven't written in a week. Was hospitalized on Thursday. I went four weeks without solid food. Every tube feeding came back up. Donna tried so hard to help me. Emotionally, she is depleted from conflicts with her daughter. We both cried on each other's shoulders for days, Donna for losing her relationship with her daughter and me the thought of losing my life.

The physical pain got to be too much. I no longer cared about my bony body or balding head. When I no longer could walk up a flight of stairs, it was bad. Wherever I am, I sit when I suddenly need to: on a curb, a bench, or a stranger's bumper. Then, in the grocery store, I collapsed.

Somehow Donna and I lost the car keys, and when we no longer could put off the hospital, we were stranded on the front steps. We both started crying. I held my bucket on my lap. I felt very close to death. I knew I had to make a decision. We called a cab instead of an ambulance. I was in and out of consciousness.

Blessed nurses at the hospital with IVs full of vitamins and nutrients, lots of pain meds, clean sheets, wonderful care! Five days to stabilize me.

Back home, all hell broke loose. Simbah attacked Donna. She spent three hours in the emergency room getting stitches and five shots. Next, Donna had a flat tire while she was using Marissa's car. Marissa and Ryan had just returned from Gainesville; they were worn out and of no help to Donna. Donna, at her wit's end, went off on them. By the time I—still in my hospital bed—heard from her, she was ready to pack it up and stay with one of my girlfriends. So wrapped up in my own misery, I felt insulted, even with the cat attack. I had nothing to give anyone.

Next day, big pow-wow around my hospital bed. Donna was insisting on going elsewhere, to Gina and Mark's, a friend's, even a hotel. I cried and said if she and the kids didn't work it out, the rift would only get bigger. Common sense prevailed, and everyone went out to breakfast the next day. Somehow they got it together to see Auntie Donna off at the airport.

Once alone again, the tension began to build between the siblings. My first night home from the hospital, Rissy flipped out and actually bit Ryan on his chest. Just like Simbah with Donna! Rissy lost control. We were all screaming at each other and crying. "I may have two weeks left, and this is how you want to remember it?" I yelled.

"Stop saying that! I can't take it!" Marissa yelled back.

Ryan lost it and threw her on the sofa, saying "We are losing our mother, you spoiled brat!"

Things deteriorated quickly; Ryan tossed Marissa's phone, and it shattered.

Then it began to thunder and lightning, followed by a downpour. Hysterical Rissy went for her car keys, but I had already hidden them. I looked at my son and daughter's tear-stained faces, and my heart broke. Yet I longed for the security and peace of my hospital bed.

The rain continued to pour down, and then we lost power. We were emotionally spent, nothing left to give each other.

* * * * *

Later that evening, Marissa came to hug me. Ryan had a few beers. We are so adrift in our sea of pain. Tomorrow, treatment begins again.

November 12, 2009
Thursday
7:00 a.m.

Walking into the chemotherapy room was like walking into a lion's den. Now my body knows what is going to happen. Involuntary shaking begins, then the alternation of hot and cold. This morning I prayed that I would totally surrender to Jesus Christ, just to give me the last eight days of courage to finish treatment. Pushing my now-skeletal self, I went into battle with a stronger will to live.

Now I feed myself easily with the tube and have mastered the sitting shower. Hip, hip, hooray!

I'm giving this last push of effort my all. I can beat this thing.

* * * * *

Every day I will say thank you for the treatment available to me. Every day is one day closer to the finish line. I have changed my lens.

Falling behind on my bills, I must find a way to do paperwork. Regardless of my fear of cancer killing me or losing the house, I refuse to waste emotion on negative thoughts. I cannot give up.

Today is the turning point. Health must be first on my list; then everything else will fall into place. Making a new battle plan, starting now! Lord, be with me every step of the way, I request.

November 13, 2009

I was lying on the sofa, feeling sad. Marissa brought a precious two-year-old little boy (she nannies part time) over to see me. She placed Joshie on my stomach. He has delayed development and eye problems. His blue eyes darted back and forth, looking at this new person lying in a heap.

Marissa said, "Josh, tell Grandmom what I taught you today." With that, he pointed to his chest and with a big smile stammered, "I Joshie."

That did it. The tears flowed and I thanked God for the incentive I prayed for. What a healing to see the pride Marissa, with her little charge, showed.

November 17, 2009

Hey, it's working! Less tears, more hope! That, plus I finally put my pain meds directly into my feeding tube. What took me so long? Why didn't anyone suggest that? I have five radiation treatments to go, and *no more chemo*! I had my last one yesterday. I am feeling okay. The vomiting has slowed down, and I have some strands of hair left. I'm down twenty-five pounds and losing daily. Didn't even know I was chubby! Walking by the full-length mirror is frightening. I see a skeletal woman with a tube dangling from her abdomen. My breasts are empty pouches, my hip bones jut out. It is not pretty. Did I really model professionally? I still was doing swimsuit modeling at fifty. I took my beautiful body for granted. Where did my butt go?

* * * * *

My rift with Donna hurts me. I'm so sad about our last visit. My friend told me that Donna told her that Dave did not call me back. He did. It just took a while. I still feel loved by him, even if he is not there for me in the way Donna would like to see.

December 23, 2009
CAT Scan

A month has gone by. All I can say is I am not the same person. First, I got through treatment. Pure hell. No words can describe it. The puking, pain, and plain stink of cancer. Toxins coming out of your pores. Nobody tells you how horrid the treatment is. If people knew, they would just opt out. Endurance is the only way to get through it. My faith was a tremendous gift. If you do not understand your own part of humanity and know your creator already suffered beyond anything we endure here, it must be very overwhelming. Even with faith and loved ones, we all have our breaking point. My heart is full of love for every kind doctor or nurse, every friend or stranger who stepped up to help me. Just knowing my kids love me and, believe it or not, feeling "chosen" by God for this assignment. Teaching empathy to others and humility to me, was, indeed, a gift from this ordeal.

A depression hit me after treatment. It was like post-partum depression, but without the joy of a baby. When I finally got it, that I could die, my faith and positive thinking took a nose dive. The realization "I'm fighting for my life," there is no polite way to say, scared me shitless.

Today I had dye put through my body. This procedure should show whether the tumors are gone. I am supposed to get the results in five days. I have turned the situation over to Jesus Christ. I honestly do not know what I will do if this treatment did not kill the cancer. Possibly, I will walk into the ocean and just let go. I am that serious; I have hit the wall.

December 27, 2009

How I am writing, I don't even know. Christmas blew up on me, and Marissa moved out.

My heart is shattered in a million pieces. I am all alone. Tomorrow is the day I find out my fate, and I have very little positive energy left to muster up my courage.

Where do I begin? Ryan was good for three weeks. He truly helped me. He kept his drinking to a minimum. His girlfriend, Julie, came and stayed with us on her way to Philly to see her family for the holidays. She was sweet, and we enjoyed four days together.

Then Jay came. I did not invite him, as I know I am too fragile to deal with his dependency issues right now. But Ryan and Marissa invited him, included their adopted brother, and I love them for embracing Jay. If I were ready to have him in my home again, I would have some pre-set boundaries. As it was, he arrived on December 23rd. His biological sister, Rachel, with toddler and husband arrived, too, from Georgia.

* * * * *

Ryan and Marissa had suggested I try medical-grade marijuana through a vaporizer for my nausea. (They would hear me up six or seven times a night, vomiting.) Of course, as an adult, I was against it. Finally one day, sick of being sick, I relented. It worked! After a total of three times, I was never sick to my stomach again. Then I understood why HIV and cancer patients lobby to legalize it.

However, once I relented, the kids interpreted that to mean they could indulge, too, to get high and chill out. They kept it in the garage, which quickly became a hang-out, complete with old sofas and music. Marissa did not, in my opinion, need this influence, and things went downhill quickly. Young people do not have the discipline or good decision-making skills necessary for a situation like this. Now I had the problem of getting this to stop, which I did quickly.

First mistake, the pot. Second mistake, giving all three adult kids at home money for Christmas. They started their own party early, and it continued on Christmas Eve day. I took Jay out shopping, trying to reestablish a bond. We went out early in the morning, me leaning on a cart for support.

Jay has been working as a chef in Gainesville and Key West and is very talented. He helped me plan three special holiday meals for fifteen people. Ryan, who also has cooked professionally for years, offered to do the cooking with Jay to help me out. Two hundred and fifty dollars later, we were done. After everything was put away or gift wrapped, I took a much-needed nap. My daughter Rachel rested with me and the baby, Lance Jr., sleeping between us.

That Afternoon

When I awoke, I began to panic about getting the Christmas Eve dinner started. I always use my best china and real silver for holidays. Under the circumstances of my illness and poor energy level, I broke down and bought Christmas paper plates and Santa Claus napkins. George and his kids arrived. Now I had nine house guests.

Apparently, Ryan and Jay hit the egg nog while I was sleeping. Not only was nothing started, they were in foul moods. Jay said he would help me after he ate something. When Jay grabbed a Christmas plate off the buffet, I said "use something else—those are for the company." He would probably have gone along with just grabbing another plate, but Ryan egged him on: "Jay, we're not good enough for the paper plates. Let's go back down into the slave quarters." Jay picked up the nasty attitude, and we all lost our tempers.

Plus, I already knew that when booze is in, brains are out. They stormed out of the room, went back downstairs, and left me hanging.

I called to Rachel to come help me get everything in the oven. When Gina and Mark came, I put them right to work. Everything was finally under control when Marissa, in a sullen mood, came home to join us. Not even the little nieces and nephews could snap her out of it. The strain was horrendous, but we made it through dinner. I had to sneak upstairs to give myself a can of formula in my feeding tube. (I'm getting really good at moving food around on my plate when I am at the table, so that others, it seems, do not notice that I am not actually eating.)

When it was time to open gifts, the boys did not come upstairs to join us. Marissa was like a statue, showing no emotion. What a letdown. I lived for this grief?

* * * * *

Christmas morning, history repeats itself. I dragged myself to the kitchen to make a nice brunch. We did the last round of gifts; Ryan and Jay boycotted Christmas, hungover.

David came over to see his sons. He told me not to wake them, and he was insulted that they were not up: "They knew I was expected." He decided to leave, another letdown.

I'll be honest. With nine house guests, it was fine with me to let them sleep it off. After David left, Ryan came upstairs like a bear! Apparently, the inside garage door got locked, and instead of just pushing the button for the automatic garage-door opener, he and Jay sat in there and stewed!

Everyone started arguing. I just wanted peace on Christmas. George tried to talk some sense into Ryan and Jay. Ryan exploded and blamed everyone in the family for his problems. Then Ryan announced he was converting to the Muslim religion, and we would not see him for fifteen years. (I believe he was having some sort of black-out as he was making no sense.) I dug up my last $100.00 to get them both bus tickets home. They packed and went off with no hugs goodbye. They left us all emotionally spent.

After a quiet day of board games and napping, everyone went to bed early. We were all sound asleep at midnight when the phones started ringing. Ryan and Jay had gotten on the wrong bus and went south instead of north. Then they lost their luggage by leaving it unattended.

This went on until 3:00 a.m. Finally, I shut my phone off. Grandson Evan came upstairs and said, "Grandmom, Dumb and Dumber are on my phone for you."

* * * * *

Meanwhile, Kendra and Marissa had a midnight curfew. Kendra made it in time, but no Marissa! I went downstairs to question Kendra about Marissa's whereabouts. After nine unanswered calls to her cell, I was a wreck. Apparently, her boyfriend sneaked her (because she was tipsy) into our house to avoid me. I had all I could do to keep my cool with Marissa slurring her words. Then she dropped a bombshell: "James is picking me up in the morning. I'm moving in with his family."

I had not even met this new boyfriend yet. But, silently, I agreed. She has to go!

The next morning a red Mustang pulls up, a very handsome young man behind the wheel. He began loading his trunk with Marissa's belongings.

In my bathrobe and barefoot, I went outside like a zombie and yelled to him: "If my daughter is moving in with you, come in the house and speak to me man to woman!"

I asked everyone else to give up privacy except for my oldest and very logical son, George. I knew I needed male back-up. Twice, Marissa appeared, saying, "James, you don't have to listen to them!"

James said, firmly, "Marissa, go wait for me."

Like a scolded child, she left. Then James announced, "I am in love with your daughter. She will be safe with me and my family." We went round and round, and he was very polite. He programmed his cell number into my phone and promised that they would keep in touch.

Marissa kissed me bye and with her sobbing her eyes out, they peeled out of the driveway. I felt like I lost three kids in twenty-four hours.

Everyone else left the next day, and here I was alone with Simbah, numb. I put the alarm on and climbed the stairs. Tomorrow I find out if I live or die. This is when a partner would be nice.

Evening

Marissa came by the house to ask for money for her car repairs. "No," I said. "Now you are an adult on your own." I also informed her that her car, medical, and dental insurance would all be cancelled. She threw a tantrum and blamed me for everything that has ever gone wrong in her life.

"Have fun alone at the doctor's," she said as she stormed out. Because I kept my cool and didn't bite, she tried the old "you don't love me" card. I stuck to my guns.

My battle with cancer has given me more strength than I ever knew I had. That and my faith have kept me somewhat sane.

January 5, 2010

Obviously, it was not good news. I have been in shock and depressed. Where do I begin? On December 28th, DeeAnn picked me up to go see Dr. Feinstein. He walked in with a poker face. Oh, shit, that must be what they teach them in medical school. I knew it was not going to be a champagne night.

He drew a breath and said, "I'm so sorry. I don't have good news. You have a malignant tumor on your voice box. It is blocking your airway. You will need surgery and lose your ability to speak or eat, for you will need a tracheotomy ASAP as you could stop breathing anytime, due to the tumor's location and obstruction. The tongue will be amputated also, as that's the location of the primary tumor."

Whatever was said after that, I have no recollection of. All I remember is walking across the parking lot with DeeAnn, arm in arm, in dead silence.

Then my cell phone rang. It was George and I burst into tears. I could not control myself. One by one, my children called, and then DeeAnn dropped me off. Sitting on my sofa with Simbah, I opened up the sealed report. There was some good news! Two stage-four tumors were gone! The one the doctor had told me about was new. I made an appointment with the ENT and also scheduled another PET scan as Dr. Feinstein had instructed.

* * * * *

The first thing the radiologist, Dr. Bushbaum, said to me was, "I had your results Christmas Eve, but I did not want to ruin your holiday." What a joke! Maybe my family would have held me instead of falling apart while waiting on pins and needles for the report.

Thinking Back to New Year's Eve
December 31, 2009

Here I am at Dr. Galin's. He's my ENT. DeeAnn took me again. When we pulled up to the hospital, I started trembling; it was reaction to the day I found out I had cancer.

He put me in that horrible plastic chair again and proceeded to put the camera through my nostrils down my throat. He said that even if it's a new tumor, it would be a three on a scale to nine. He also told me he has seen many false reports due to scar tissue appearing to be tumors on the scans. He also disagreed with the oncologist and radiologist about my airway being blocked. He gave me hope! He said if it were as bad as the other two doctors thought, I would not be sitting there breathing on my own.

With new hope, I called my son George and got the name of a world-renowned Russian specialist, Dr. Vaysberg, at George's hospital, Shands at the University of Florida. I needed a second opinion before I gave up my tongue and voice box. If he agrees with the first two doctors that I need major surgery, I am frightened to my core. They would cut me ear to ear.

January 11, 2010

I drove four hours, alone, up to George's in Gainesville. On car trips, I usually sing along to my favorite CDs. I soon found out I had lost that ability.

George gave me his master bedroom and bath; it meant so much to me as I needed a private spot, like a breast-feeding mom, for my feeding tube. Took my meds and settled in my son's comfortable bedroom. I looked over to his dresser, and there was a picture of me and another of my mom in two small frames on each side of his Buddha. It gave me such comfort to see his little setup. He loves me!

January 12, 2010
Tuesday

Praise Jesus! The Shands' specialist did every test imaginable on me yesterday, and no tumor could be found!

I am in a state of shock. Prayer works, and I am spared.

Drove the five hours home on pure adrenaline. I am wiped out but truly happy. For now, no surgery.

January 17, 2010
Sunday

Feeling a tiny bit better day by day. I am still using the feeding tube but eating a little soup and mushy foods.

Tomorrow, I am supposed to get my full Shands' report. They may tell me I need two lymph nodes removed, if they are suspicious. No problem. I can live without them if I need to. As long as I can keep my tongue and voice box, I'm a happy camper.

Today my friend Maria and her husband, Paul, took Marissa and me to see *Phantom of the Opera* in Fort Lauderdale. It was our Christmas gift. We got all dolled up. I wore hair extensions and borrowed a size two cocktail dress. We went to dinner and I managed a bowl of soup. My whole body was crying for my bed, but I enjoyed knowing that this treat was their way of saying "we knew you would be alive" to enjoy the play.

Marissa decided to move back home, and things are much calmer between us. Ryan and I had met for breakfast in Gainesville on my way out of town. He has a new job! He also went into therapy. All positive news! We had a healing visit.

I'm still trying to get my weight up to 120. At 125, the tube can come out!

Working a few hours a day, and trying to save the little bit of hair I have left. As long as the cancer stays gone, I am embracing my life. I will live life fully and forever be grateful for whatever gift of time I am granted.

Last night Gina and Mark asked me to join them and the kids at an ice cream parlor. Just to sit outdoors on a breezy South Florida night eating an ice cream cone was such a blessing. One month ago I was a stinking heap on my bed, vomiting all night. Now I am so grateful to God.

January 18, 2010
Monday

No results yet. Back to the waiting game. I phoned my ENT to see if anyone had the report yet; a recording said the office was closed for MLK Day. Yikes! Could someone please let me know if I am in remission?!

David called me tonight to see how I was doing. He then shared changes about his own health issues. It was a comforting call.

Marissa's boyfriend called me to check in, and his family sent some Peruvian tea over to help detox my body. Everyone has been so kind to me.

January 19, 2010
Tuesday

No news yet! I started phoning the hospital at 8:00 a.m. and did not give up until 4:00 p.m. I kept my phone in my pocket all day.

Finally, I got a person! A very nice nurse told me my report was done but not entered into the computer yet. Desperate to hear the formal report, I had no choice to wait it out. I cannot plan a future until I know I have one.

January 20, 2010

Still no news!! Now I'm getting cranky. No call back from the M. D. I got through to the hospital at 3:00 p.m. They told me he had eight more patients to see before he answered any calls. What are the odds he will call tonight with that schedule?

Ryan, Rachel, and Jay all called me to check in. Every time the phone rings, I jump. Please, please, please God, give me good news.

Marissa and James are holed up downstairs eating pizza. I can smell it, but I am holed up in my room with a can of formula. Yum! Just wishing I will be able to have a slice of pizza again someday.

January 22, 2010
Friday

Still waiting! I have not received any formal results yet. I am feeling very queasy. What I did find out is that the chief of radiology has not had time to finish his full report. Last night, George called me from Connecticut. My granddaughter Kendra is checking out the officers training program with the U. S. Coast Guard. I am so proud of her. When we spoke, I asked George if he had ever met this chief of radiology. Just so happens they are on a committee together. I asked George to pull some strings to speed things up. He promised to call him.

Tomorrow, a group of inspectors is coming to my townhouse to open the walls to verify whether or not I have Chinese drywall. I am curious if this contributed to my head and neck cancer.

* * * * *

Life is strange. I have a dinner date! My friend Doreen has a dear friend, Ray, in town who shares my diagnosis. How weird is that; we can chat about our stomach tubes, if nothing else.

We went to a very nice restaurant, Bonefish. It was a joy to be among the living, having fun. I even bought some new pants. Size four, still hanging off me. Ray was a nice man, but Doreen's boyfriend was more my type, darn it!

Back online at 3:00 a.m., where I read that some people get two good years after stage-four cancer. Then it returns elsewhere. TMI (too much information).

January 26, 2010
Tuesday

Finally! News. I have one suspicious lymph node that will need another PET scan. Otherwise, things look good. I asked if I was in remission, and they said I cannot use that word for two years!

Should I feel joy yet? I'm frozen. I only told two people so far. My prayers are answered, but I need to quickly figure out what I do with this time I have been granted. Short or long, it is a pure gift.

January 27, 2010
Wednesday

Other than Marissa and George, I have not made all the calls to family and friends yet. This feeling of being overwhelmed is immobilizing me. It is as if the governor just put my execution on hold.

First person to mend my relationship with is Rissy. After three or four calls, I am beat. Laying on my bed watching PBS with Simbah purring beside me. I am on idle.

My mind is reviewing the past few months. Losing Jane, my boss, to ovarian cancer; my treatment; family blow-ups. I need quiet time to process everything.

Thank you, God, for a second chance at life.

January 28, 2010

Today I am back at the oncologist; blood counts are not good. Still dropping weight and hair. Dr. Feinstein reminded me once again not to use the word *remission*. He droned on about the suspicious node, and I just felt deflated.

Trying to do normal errands is so difficult. A 3:00 p.m. meeting at work pushed me to my limit. Now it is 7:00 p.m., and I'm in bed. Marissa had a date. I feel lonely and sad tonight.

January 29, 2010
Friday

Woke up very sick with a disgusting peg tube back-up. Had to pull myself together for a work lunch/meeting. It was supposed to be a celebration of my co-worker Larry becoming my boss. Maria and Larry had beautiful surf and turf salads, hot rolls, and French fries. I pretended to eat my soup, but it would not go down. I wore a loose dress to hide the peg tube. Pretending to feel okay, so as not to bring everyone's mood down is so much work!

Later in the day, I bought Marissa some groceries so she would have a decent meal after working at the spa today. Can't join her. No appetite at all. And cannot taste anything. For the first time in my life, I am constipated. Now I'm so thin that naked, I look like a starvation victim. It is horrible to face. I do *want* to live! I can't suffer any more. My faith is all that's keeping me going.

January 30, 2010
Saturday morning

Finally figured out I can pour prune juice directly into my peg-tube! Eight full ounces at bedtime. No horrid taste. Why wouldn't the nurses suggest this to me before? There is a manual for my dryer and my toaster, but not for my cancer.

January 31, 2010
Sunday

After no solid food for three months, it took a lot to jumpstart my body. Always blessed with a fast metabolism, it was shocking to have my body shut down. Just using the bathroom is a blessing! My heart breaks for all the people in nursing homes that this happens to.

One more PET scan—for the suspicious lymph node—to go. Sometimes a sadness comes over me, survivor's guilt. I think of my friend Jane; why am I still here? Now it's a good day, bad day erratic roller coaster.

By the grace of God, I'm still here and June, my former boss, is not. Why? I don't know. I continue to think about this strange twist of fate. It does make me feel that I should be very gracious and thankful. I hope I can be kinder and less driven.

Still daydreaming about having one last life partner. Dear friend Robert calls, but he still has his "snowbird" girlfriend. David calls, but he has had twenty years to make amends with me and has not. What make me think my battle with cancer would soften his heart?

I want to resume some kind of life but only if I know I am going to live. Tired, hungry, and lonely. I'm back at the bottom of the mountain.

February 2, 2010
Tuesday

I was scheduled at work today at 11:30 a.m. Time to pick up my prescription and the dress—the one I had borrowed for the play—from the cleaners. Feeling semi-normal, I thought it would be a nice gesture to pick up Spanish pastries for my coworkers. Next, I ran into the grocery store to send Ryan and his girlfriend a Western Union gift certificate, then the post office, and, lastly, I returned to the market for some cream for the coffee at work.

My arms were full of newspapers, cream, and whatever else I thought we needed when a little old lady started freaking out. She had lost her grocery list. "Can you please help me?" she asked, obviously in a panic. I turned on my heels to look in back of where I was standing and slipped and lost my footing. I began to stumble forward and, instead of dropping the contents of my arms, I hung on tight and crashed into a canned-goods display, stopping only when my nose cracked into the hard wooden bin. Then I blacked out.

When I regained consciousness, four EMTs were hovering over me; a crowd of gawkers surrounded us. A tiny little girl with a head full of braids came over to me and bent down. "Here's my lucky penny," she said, and put a penny in my hand.

So ashamed of myself sprawled on the floor, I refused to go in the ambulance. Feeling old and weak, right there on that dirty floor, I began to sob. Once again, I literally hit bottom.

* * * * *

I showed up for work late, with the start of two shiners. My face was so swollen, they made me leave early. Marissa was upset to see me banged up and was kind to me. She gave me a shoulder massage, so at least something positive came from this.

I now look like I went a round with Rocky.

February 5, 2010
Friday

Five days later, my eyes are still black and blue. It is humiliating. The Chinese-drywall inspector showed up and asked "what does the other guy look like?"

Decided to ask DeeAnn over for tea. After she left, I did a little housework, then read and napped. Even with all my problems, life is still good.

February 27, 2010
Sunday morning

"Further and quicker" said Pastor Joel Osteen today on his TV sermon. It was the first thing that fed my soul in the three weeks since I wrote.

Shands finally called me with good news: "no sign of cancer left anywhere"!

Just when I was about to jump for joy, my oncologist called and said it could recur anytime for the next two years. I must go monthly for blood work and to the ENT for scopes.

Of course I will do as directed; I am so thrilled. The pain has subsided, and I am eating a little soft food. I still cannot taste anything, but I can smell and I remember what was good. My saliva production did not return, and the dry mouth is a horrible thing. I carry my sprays and special gels along with my water jug every-where I go.

I'm learning to sip broth with everything I try to eat, and I'm now under 112 pounds. My size four clothes fall off me. I still have my stomach tube, and unless I can get up to 125, it is not going any-where. I have new wrinkles on my once-pretty face. My firm, cellu-lite-free legs are now two sticks. If I catch sight of myself walking by a mirror, it looks like someone let the air out of me. I took for granted rounded curves and nice skin. My once pink nipples are now burnt raisins from the radiation. Funny, some women would be happy to have this body. But I was spoiled and took mine for granted. I'm alive; I'll take whatever I have!

* * * * *

It is so difficult to get through a full day of work because my en-ergy level and ability to focus are so low. I need to nap but do not want to ask for any special treatment, so I just keep pushing. My survival occupies my mind. My substitute is still helping me out, thank God. Maria has been a blessing.

I will never be a workaholic again. Slowly, I have learned I need to tune into myself—body, mind, and, most importantly, spirit. Sometimes, for instance, when Marissa gives me a hard time, I have a fleeting thought that "I don't want to live like this." Just as quickly, I visualize my cells dividing and multiplying. I pray that negative thoughts have not allowed any new cancer cells to take root.

Yesterday, I went by myself to look at a little apartment on the Intracoastal. It has lush trails and a private beach and dock. (It used to be the mansion of Al Capone!) If I decide to move, it will be alone. Marissa's boyfriend, James, is now under my roof every night. While he seems to be a nice guy, I cannot go to my own kitchen without a bra on without running into him looking into the fridge. When he is in a towel, it is, as the kids say, "Awkward."

* * * * *

Marissa gave me a hug when I got my good news. Hooray. At eighteen years old, it is still all about her. Her car broke down two weeks ago. I have tried to have it fixed, picked up the tab for towing, and shared my car. All to no avail. She continues to whine about no wheels. She is not understanding that I cannot snap my fingers and buy her a new car. Her sense of entitlement is not easy to live with.

Yesterday, I sat Marissa and James down. I explained that if I move out, you are on your own: utilities, car insurance, food, gas, everything. (I have been covering most of the expenses.)

"Why can't you stay and treat the situation as three working adults?" was their response. Problem is, two of them have never bought laundry detergent or milk or returned my car with a full tank of gas. Also, I have been holed up in my bedroom for privacy. There is no more freedom in my own home. The kids use the townhouse like a hotel. There is always a pile of dirty towels, dishes in the sink, and the smell of pot. Empty glasses are on the patio, and they do not respect my rules. At eighteen and twenty, they are pushing the limits. The cord must be cut and soon!

* * * * *

Last night, my phone rang at 2:00 a.m. My ex-husband (from my teenage years), who I have not seen or heard from in over forty years, chose to wake me out of a deep sleep to say "hey." He was the same self-centered jerk He saw online that I was "ill" and because he is a night owl, he said, he went ahead and called, even though it was late.

Who in their right mind calls at 2:00 a.m. a person recovering from stage-four cancer? I guess he was bored or restless or something. He kept saying "your voice is so different." No shit, Shakespeare, I was nineteen the last time we spoke, and my throat has had a little bit of a rough run lately. "No hard feelings, right?" is how he ended the call.

So, here I finally had the chance to say something to him, after my family had disowned me over him—he was West Indian and it was 1968—and I had one baby with him and one on the way when he walked out of our lives forever. What did I say? "No problem. Thanks for calling."

* * * * *

Coming full circle, I know how I want to live. Peace is everything. Without health, there is no peace. So that is number one. The day-to-day battles with Marissa over stupid, petty things have got to end. Wear the thong with the short skirt, daughter; it is your body and your decision. Pierce, tattoo, have a ball. I did my best for almost nineteen years. I deserve peace. This is not a decision. It is mandatory for my survival.

The same way people relapse into alcohol or drug addiction—that is the way I am looking at my cancer recovery. I must "detach with kindness," as Al-anon teaches.

Slowly, I erase the signs of sickness from the house. Bottles of pills, cases of formula, tubes and funnels, all the cancer binders full of prescription instructions and medical paperwork: out of every room, everywhere. I am trying to *not* see what reminds me of being the patient. My self-perception is no longer that of a sick person. All my good clothes, suits and beautiful dresses, slacks, blouses, everything that does not fit me anymore went to my daughter Gina.

It is better to have a handful of size twos then a rack full of clothes that remind me of the cancer.

As I weed out the excess from my life, I become calmer and more self-aware. I know what matters to me. My comfortable bed with my hand-stitched quilt made just for me by my sister Donna gives me peace. A few sentimental things from the kids and grandkids, my favorite books beside me. All the rest I have been giving away. Nothing makes you clean out the clutter like a brush with death. Who wants to leave their personal crap for the family to sift through? I certainly do not.

* * * * *

My red-headed buddy Simbah went to heaven last Thursday night. He continued to attack family and friends randomly and unprovoked. When I was up at George's to see the specialist, I came home to Marissa a bloody mess from one of Simbah's attacks.

Yes, Simbah sat beside me all those weeks giving me comfort, and he was my buddy for seven years. When I got sick, he only loved me. He became so angry and unpredictable; the decision had to be made.

I had become like those pit-bull owners who justify every attack as the children or victim's fault.

So on a rainy, miserable night, Marissa and I drove Simbah to animal control headquarters. We cried our eyes out in the pouring rain. I did realize, however, that I would never forgive myself if Simbah continued the attacks that had already hurt others.

I had called Dr. Craig as my friend, therapist, and fellow animal lover. After I spilled out the facts, he said, calmly, "It is time."

The cancer battle gave me the strength to follow through and do what I had to do. Losing a pet used to put me in a depression for weeks. Now it hurts, of course, but I see it as part of life. I am here. He is gone. It will be okay.

* * * * *

I am still on the mild anti-depressant; thank God I gave in and started taking it. It was another tiny bit of help. Still taking the thyroid medicine faithfully. The doctor questioned why I was still losing my hair after chemo ended. Also the pounds kept dropping. Now I do a comb-over across the top of my head and wear a padded bra. That's okay! I am alive!

Oh! I can read again! I am back to two-to-three books a week. What a thrill. Also my magazine and newspaper addictions are once again giving me daily pleasure.

My faith was tested, but it is still strong. I am looking forward to the day I can say thank you to God for the cancer, that it was worth the growth and awareness. Still too raw. Still too soon to go there.

* * * * *

Never will I be the same. I did not know how much I needed

friends. Every card, every lovely note, every visit or call meant the world to me. My work buddies Sandi and Heidi's constant prayers fed my soul. Just to walk to the mailbox and find it full of cards, medals of saints, and even fruit cake was a daily blessing that lifted my spirits. My home had fresh flowers and the goodness of people displayed everywhere.

For too long, I was an island with blinders on. God knocked me on my butt. For me to be able to say "I need people" is my gift. Everyone knew I was reclusive, but now I see I was really selfish. As much as I love solitude, I have opened the door to others. I have the grandkids over more. So what if they wreck the house? I accept more invitations, go out more often, and get out of my comfort zone. My life lesson is that nothing bad happens out there. I can even have fun. And my sofa and books are waiting for me when I come home. Since my diagnosis, I say "yes" more often.

When I sat in all the waiting rooms at all the different treatment facilities, I had time to observe the married couples waiting together. It hit home. Being part of a couple means so much. Yes, you give up your privacy and space, but you may gain a best friend to hold you when you are frightened to death.

Yes, friends and some family step up, but at night when you wake up every hour to vomit and your are on your knees begging God to just get you through until the sun comes up, those physical arms are missed.

* * * * *

Did the Chinese drywall give me cancer? I don't know. Staying in this townhouse is not good for my health. As I have been notified by the health department and my doctors, I must leave. I will have to walk away from my home that I worked so hard to buy on my own. It is not saleable and now way below the $200,000 still mort-gaged. My Toyota was just recalled, so I am also stuck with a car that cannot be traded in. Home and car worthless.

My eighteen-year-old daughter is still making gray what strands of hair I have left. My beloved Simbah, dead.

And, yet, I am still happy! I am alive, and the pain has subsided! Life is about what we cannot see: health, loyalty, love, faith, and other intangibles. Now I understand deeply those two Bible vers-es I always liked: "This is a life of faith, not sight, for whatever is visible is temporary. We know our suffering is temporary. What is not seen is forever."

March 7, 2010

It is Sunday morning and the police just left. Marissa's boyfriend got all macho and stuck his nose in our mother-daughter spat. When he raised his voice and got in my face, I dialed 911.

He is gone. He is not allowed on our development's property. I am very sad about it, but he crossed a line. I am healthy enough to draw boundaries to protect us. Marissa went after him, but quickly came back and apologized. She lay beside me face-to-face on the sofa. It was our first real body hug since my diagnosis. Her body was racked with sobs and tears streamed down our faces. I held her tightly. We fell asleep in each other's arms, just like when she was still my baby.

March 8, 2010

The hormones prevailed. Today Marissa decided to pack her

things, once again, and move in with her boyfriend's family. Her choice, not mine.

So here I am, alone again. No mate, no kids, no cat. That is okay. *I am alive*!

Life's problems will always be around, but most problems are not unsolvable.

Nothing compares to cancer.

Money worries, kid and work stress, it is all part of life. Do I feel a sadness to be in the midst of all this turmoil? Yes, but I am currently cancer free! There is a joy deep down in my soul that no one can take from me.

"Now you saved me," I cry out to God, "please reveal to me the reason!" Surely it is not just to work and muddle through life's problems. Shortly, my prayers will be answered, I know, and once again will prove that our heavenly father knows our needs better than we know ourselves or even our own desires.

March 10, 2012

Life is back on track. Rachel called for me to wire her and her family money to get through a rough spot. I send what I can.

Marissa's car broke down, and I pulled some strings; a good friend helped us out, just for the cost of parts.

Gina came by for a visit yesterday; we laughed over a cup of tea. It feels wonderful to have that relationship whole again.

Life is short and precious. I will never be an island again. I need people, friends, and my family.

* * * *

Many times I think back to November and December, just lying on the sofa in pure agony, with my disgusting puke bucket by my side. Just praying to get through it, minute by minute. As rough as life can be, it is pretty damn good.

March 12, 2012

Tomorrow I go in for my first blood work since anyone whispered "possible remission."

My relationships continue to heal and grow. Dear friends have shown such compassion on my darkest days. My faith remains strong.

God willing, I will be a part of the lives of my children and grandbabies a little longer.

I slowly get back to teaching and rush home to nap as my body still repairs. Some co-workers look at me like I am the walking dead. I think my illness was too close for comfort. People have to face their own mortality in their own time, I suppose.

As the hair and weight slowly return, I feel the wonder of anticipation of what God has for me.

March 18, 2010

Hung over! How could I be so stupid to think I could go to a St. Patrick's Day happy- hour party and indulge? I felt pretty and happy for the first time in a long time, and I had so much fun. However, the smaller, still recovering body could not handle any alcohol. Note to self—do not go from canned formula to alcohol, especially as a size two.

Still, I must get to work today. My head hurts, and I am ashamed of myself for abusing my health this way. Popping two aspirin, I cry out to God again: "Surely you did not spare me for this. Please reveal to me my purpose. Why am I still here?"

* * * * *

Walking onto campus, I take in the beauty. Did they always have this lush landscaping and so many fountains? Everything seems so bright and beautiful.

As I walk into my department, a student I know slightly walks right up to me. "Ms. Barbee, I hear you love children and had a bunch. Would you be interested in mentoring a little girl, ten years old? She has been in and out of shelters and foster care. Her dad is in jail. Her mom does drugs and dropped her off with my husband and me over a year ago. We have our hands full with five children, including one-year-old twins."

"Yes," I hear myself saying. No questions. I just knew I had to be open to hear my destiny, what God had in store for me.

"I can pick her up Saturday," I said, "and take her for ice cream. Just give me the address."

* * * * *

Fast forward to Saturday. I had phoned Marissa and told her I was going to meet a kid from the shelter who got left off with an overwhelmed family. "Mom," she said, "you are old and sick. What are you thinking?"

"I am thinking," I said, "that I still have something to give, and God willing, I will be here a while longer."

As I drive to Delray, I am nervous as I look up and down streets for the address. Ah. There it is, plastic toys scattered all over the front yard.

I pull up and get out. Three or four men are dismantling an engine in the driveway and having some beer. As I introduce myself, I see twin girls in saggy diapers playing in the dirt. A beautiful curly-headed boy runs around with a sharp stick. A thin, little girl, brunette, looking sad, quiet as a mouse, sits on the front step.

The men look over and stop speaking Spanish. All of a sudden, I feel like I may seem to be someone from Children's Protective Services. Quickly, I explain that I am here to take the "foster child" out for a visit and that I teach at the college the mom attends. Everyone looks relieved.

The husband goes in to get his wife, and I sat myself on a wooden swing hanging from a tree. Every emotion is going through me. Am I up for this? Is that the little girl? She seems so withdrawn. Nobody speaks to me. Twice, I jump up to pull a twin from daring into the road. Just as I am wishing I had gone to Barnes and Noble instead, a beautiful blonde girl walks out of the house with the student, who says to me, "This is Destiny."

We look each other over, head to toe. She sits beside me on the swing. Her eyes are crystal blue, the sun shines on her flowing hair, and I am stunned by her healthy beauty.

"Destiny," I say, showing my surprise, I am sure, "you are a beautiful girl!" I kind of expected a ragamuffin.

"Well," she answers, "so are you. I thought you were going to be an old, fat, gray-haired lady." We both laughed.

We just continued to take each other in. Then I said, "Well, do you want to get to know me, maybe go have an ice cream? When you feel comfortable, we could go out to dinner sometime."

She looks at the peasant skirt I have on and says, "I have a skirt that looks like that. Give me a minute to go put it on. I don't have a shy bone in my body. Let's go out to dinner today!"

* * * * *

Marissa called first thing in the morning. "Well, Mom, how did it go with the kid?"

"Marissa, it was the best dinner date I've had in years. We sat by the ocean, had steaks, and laughed our heads off. I hope you can meet her next weekend when we do a sleepover."

"What are you thinking, Mom!" Marissa gasped. "I'm worried about your health."

"Just meet her," I said. "And stay open-minded, okay? Oh, and, by the way, she looks like she could be your little sister."

Postscript

Fast forward two and a half years. I am the mother of a twelve-year-old girl. It astounds me that God blessed me with another child at this stage of life.

Feeling healthy, in remission, shapely again, with a head of pretty hair.

Every sunrise is a gift. Before my feet hit the floor, I say my thanks for all the gifts: no pain, the ability to eat, feeling rested, looking forward to a cup of coffee. Peeking in on a sleepy little girl with sun-streaked hair on her pillow, teddy bear clutched in her arm. How lucky am I?

"Work" is just "work." The only joy there is the human connection with my students. Otherwise, it is just a paycheck.

I saw the redwoods in California this summer, got tanned, hiked with my Ryan, Marissa, Destiny, and my grandson Evan. Marissa and Destiny bonded as sisters. Then I even got to share a kiss or two with someone. Music is sweeter. Food is better, even with no taste buds or saliva. Texture, smell, and sharing the experience is worth it.

All the kids, after all that worry, have grown into good adults. And guess what? David and I have a renewed relationship.

There is always hope. There is always another way out. When we trust that God has it under control, we can just get our life lessons and feel secure. The rest will fall into place.

I do not fear death. I just celebrate life.

Acknowledgments

Special thanks to DeeAnn Hoffman and Donna Chase.

Thanks to all my children and grandchildren and siblings and ex-husbands, Dave and Rich.

Thanks also to Maria and Paul, Heidi and Paul, Debra, Dr. Craig, Blanca, Jahira, Don Kauts, Ellen, Diane and Bob, Uncle Geno, Robert, Jim, Nurse Terri, Dr. Galin, Dr. Feinstein, Dr. Buschbaum, Dr. Vaysberg, Dr. Del Negro, Nurse Dorothy, Palmaire, Freddie, Lisa and Nancy, Green Acres Christian School and EBD Ministries, Sam P., Sandi and Gary and Ms. Mae, Ann Marie, Laura, Emily, Joe and Cynthia, Doreen, Ray, Alex D., Dan and Lani, Jadira and Louise, Leta and Shayntra, Delores P., Janet D., Bette B., Patricia, Brooke, Niece Angela, Marie, Marion H., Jeanine B., Jill, Betty and Frannie, and Alan K.

And thanks to–and in loving memory of–Mark Dragula, Jane Hastings, Lauren Garcia, Stacey Fuller, Debra Sikora Selvaggio Hurt, Nathaniel Parks, and all our loved ones who have gone before us.

About My Kids

George

My oldest, George, was always an old soul. He was such an easy baby. Then, as a child, I did not have to worry he would ever forget his mittens or backpack. He could read at four and had the same level-headed common sense he still has as a man. Because he is so easy to be around, everyone accused me of him being the "favorite."

For the others, he was "a hard act to follow." His road to success was planned out: air force, then college and career and the best dad ever. Looking like he should be on the cover of *G. Q.* didn't hurt, either. How I did it at nineteen, I haven't a clue. Just good genes, I guess.

Gina

Gina was a quiet, sensitive little girl. I was probably too overbearing for her personality. She danced for years, as graceful as a swan. She was a beauty and modeled through high school. Then one day she up and quit, left with an audience awaiting a top fashion show. She let me know it was my dream, not hers, and she never looked back.

I wish I could have been more nurturing and softer for her. I was only twenty and expecting her when her dad left me. We have our issues.

Ryan

Ryan David, my one biological child with David, was my outdoor, golden, nature boy. We bonded over hikes in the woods on the coast of Maine. The older two were city kids for sure, but Ryan, ever since he was a toddler, had an appreciation for every living thing. He camped and fished in summer, snowboarded and skied like a pro in winter.

Ry's passion for life had a flip side. His intensity for life made him more vulnerable to every human emotion, and he could be a handful, especially in the temper department. When his dad had his mid-life crisis, Ryan was at the sensitive age of fourteen. I think his dad's crisis rocked his world in a negative way. He is now an organic farmer in the California mountains and a wonderfully creative chef.

Rachel

I met Rachel through Catholic Social Services when she was ten. She looked the most like me, fair and hazel eyed. What a spit fire! She navigated foster homes and keeping her little brother Jay safe all her life. She had a street-smart attitude and this saved the both of them. Once, when they were still with their biological mom, they were left home alone, and their apartment caught fire. The *Boston Globe* reported that Rachel, only six years old, stood on a chair to reach her baby brother in his crib, lifted him out, and ran outside to get them both to safety.

Rachel's defenses were always up and even when she had a calm, secure home, you couldn't get the "fight" out of her. As much trouble as Rachel caused me, she was my mini-me. Feisty, strong, and ready to take on the world. To this day, she is always upbeat and joyful: what a gift! She lives with her husband and son in Georgia.

Jay

Jay, also from Catholic Social Services, was the little boy with a head full of curls who won my heart when he was seven. How can you not open up to an adorable, sweet child who knew nothing of kindness and family life?

The day the social workers introduced Jay to Dave and me, we took him out for an ice cream. It never took much to make him happy! He was almost too good, and our family therapist warned me that the sweet, quiet ones often have a "delay of painful emotions," but I never truly realized that trauma of the first seven years would resurface someday. If only I could fix the broken pieces. A talented chef and musician, he has so much to give the world. He is expecting his first son this year.

Marissa

God gave me Marissa, my one biological child with Richard, to heal my heart from my divorce from David. The joy that ten-pound baby girl gave me saved me from myself. We were inseparable. She had me to herself once the other kids grew up and her dad and I split up. I tried to give her every experience possible, boating and adventuring together. We lived the island life in Key West. We showered outdoors by the hibiscus, we skinny-dipped in our pool and the ocean. We went out to sea on a coast guard cutter, slept under the stars at Fort Jefferson. We even re-enacted Revolutionary-era history in costume!

We were probably too close. She was in my bed until puberty, and then she decided to become her own person. When you have a baby late—I was forty-one when she was born—sometimes the line between parent and over-indulgent grandparent is quite blurred.

I didn't mean to be so selfish with her; it probably wasn't fair to her to feel "joined at the hip" with her mother. Thankfully, the cord was cut rather abruptly by my diagnosis. She is a licensed esthetician who lives with her boyfriend.

Destiny

How Destiny came into my life is covered in my journal, but I would like to say that three years have passed, and I know that she is the reason God kept me here. She is blossoming into a great spirit. She embraces all her siblings and family life.

www.ingramcontent.com/pod-product-compliance
Lightning Source LLC
Chambersburg PA
CBHW030025290326
41934CB00005B/484